To Christin
All a [illegible]
Brian

Great Teeth for Life

The Secret to a Lifetime of Good Dental Health

Brian Halvorsen, BDS, LDS RCS

iUniverse, Inc.
New York   Bloomington

Copyright © 2010 by Brian Halvorsen, BDS, LDS RCS

All rights reserved. No part of this book may be used or reproduced by any means, graphic, electronic, or mechanical, including photocopying, recording, taping or by any information storage retrieval system without the written permission of the publisher except in the case of brief quotations embodied in critical articles and reviews.

iUniverse books may be ordered through booksellers or by contacting:

iUniverse
1663 Liberty Drive
Bloomington, IN 47403
www.iuniverse.com
1-800-Authors (1-800-288-4677)

Because of the dynamic nature of the Internet, any Web addresses or links contained in this book may have changed since publication and may no longer be valid. The views expressed in this work are solely those of the author and do not necessarily reflect the views of the publisher, and the publisher hereby disclaims any responsibility for them.

ISBN: 978-1-4502-0069-1 (sc)
ISBN: 978-1-4502-0071-4 (hc)
ISBN: 978-1-4502-0070-7 (ebook)

Printed in the United States of America

iUniverse rev. date: 02/24/2010

About the Author

Brian Halvorsen is a holistic dental practitioner in Buckinghamshire, England. He founded the Prestwood Dental Health Centre in 1977. Author of *The Natural Dentist* in 1986, Brian helped found the Dental Nutrition Society and the International Academy of Oral Medicine and Toxicology (IAOMT). A member of the British Dental Association, fellow of the Royal Society of Medicine, and council member of the Dental Practitioners Association, Brian has been actively involved within the profession for thirty-five years.

When the PDH Centre was founded in 1977, Brian established the principles of prevention, and he has always worked with dental hygienists and dental health educators. In the early eighties, Brian's concern turned to holistic dentistry and the effects of materials that were currently being used, and his practice became "amalgam free" in 1985. With the advancement of cosmetic dentistry as well as adhesive dentistry, Brian saw the opportunity to work with nontoxic materials with less tooth destruction (non-reduction veneers, ceramic crowns, and composite bonding).

Cofounder of the world's first satellite TV channel dedicated to postgraduate dental education, Brian gained insight into, and knowledge of, global trends in dentistry and medicine, realizing that the future of holistic dentistry can profoundly improve the quality of many patients' lives.

Brian has lectured to dentists, medical doctors, health practitioners, and the public on the subject of this book, and he sees the importance of complete holistic care, i.e., that which encompasses *mind*, *body*, and *soul*.

To those who have suffered through lack of knowledge

Contents

About the Author	v
Special Thanks to the Following:	xiii
Foreword	xv
Introduction	xvii
Great Teeth for Life	xvii
Advice for My Readers	xvii
CHAPTER ONE	1
Why Should You Read This Book?	1
The Answer?	7
CHAPTER TWO	9
The Evolution of Dentistry: The Good, the Bad, and the Ugly	9
In the Beginning	9
Dentistry in Antiquity	12
Dentistry in the Middle Ages	14
The Beginnings of Modern Dentistry	19
Dentistry As a Profession	23
Conservative Dentistry	26
Education and Prevention	26
CHAPTER THREE	27
Teeth and Jaws: Get to Know This Vital Part of Your Body	27
The Teeth	27
The Structure of a Tooth	29
Calcification	33
Nutrition and Calcification	38
The Jaw	42
Shaping of the Jaws	44
CHAPTER FOUR	49
You Are What You Eat—and What Your Parents Ate Too!	49
Preconceptual Care	49
Postnatal Care	66
Breastfeeding	67
Maternal Diet during Lactation	69
Teething	70
Chronology of the Deciduous Teeth	71
Chronology of the Permanent Teeth	71

Moving on from Breast Milk Alone	73
Deciduous Teeth and the Dentist	81
Permanent Teeth	93
Wisdom Teeth	94
CHAPTER FIVE	**95**
Tooth Decay—Sweet Tooth/Rotten Tooth!	**95**
The Role of Sugar in Tooth Decay	96
The Progression of Tooth Decay	104
CHAPTER SIX	**114**
What's All the Fuss about Fluoride?	**114**
Fluorine	114
Dosage and the Effects on Teeth	115
Fluoride and Tooth Decay	116
Systemic Fluorides	117
Fluoridation of Water Supplies	117
Topical Fluorides	119
Fluoride Toothpastes	120
Fluoride Gels	120
Fluoride Mouth Rinses/Mouthwashes	121
CHAPTER SEVEN	**122**
Gum Disease—What Lies Beneath?	**122**
Gums	123
Causes of Gum Disease	123
Types of Periodontal Disease	128
The Signs of Gum Disease	129
The Progress of Gum Disease	133
Additional Mouth Conditions	134
A Review of Nutrition's Impact on Gum Disease	135
Dietary Supplements	136
The Role of the Dentist	137
CHAPTER EIGHT	**138**
Oral Hygiene: Ignore Your Teeth and Gums— and They Will Go Away!	**138**
Tooth Brushing	138
How to Brush Your Teeth	139
Toothbrushes	140
Electric Toothbrushes	143

Effectiveness	143
Toothpaste	144
Flossing	156
Disclosing Tablets	159
Mouthwashes	159
Toothpicks and Wood Points	160
In Conclusion	160
CHAPTER NINE	**162**
Going to the Dentist: And You Thought It Was Just about Your Teeth!	162
Dental Examinations	163
CHAPTER TEN	**172**
Stress, Stress, Stress, Stress—Four Reasons Why You Are Ill	172
Stresses That Cause Disease	173
Environmental	173
Psychological	175
Physical	177
Nutritional	179
Stress and Disease	180
Dentistry and physical stress	181
CHAPTER ELEVEN	**184**
The Importance of Good Nutrition: Feed Your Mouth, Feed Your Body	184
Diet Sheet (include quantities/weights)	185
Dietary Guidelines	187
Planning Your Healthy Diet	191
Steps toward Healthier Eating	192
CHAPTER TWELVE	**197**
Nutrition and Ageing: Detox Your Teeth and Your Body	197
The Bad News	197
The Good News	201
Dr. Brian's Diet to Reduce Your Intake of Toxins/Heavy Metals:	201
Supplements—a Twenty-First-Century Way to Avoid the Diseases of Ageing?	204
Conclusion	207
Where Do I See the Future of Holistic Dentistry/Medicine?	207

FURTHER READING 209
    Advice to the Reader 209
    Selected Bibliography from the 1986 Book
    The Natural Dentist 209
    Additional References for Great Teeth for Life 211
Beyond Diet and Lifestyle 213
    Why Supplements Are an Essential Part of the Detoxification Process 213
    Additional Reading 227
Index 229

Special Thanks to the Following:

British Dental Association Museum, Rachel Bairstow in particular, for providing and allowing me to use the historical images

Price-Pottenger Nutrition Foundation, and Joan Grinzi in particular, for their photos.

My wife, Lyn, for her love and inspiration

Ben and Adam

The editors at iUniverse

Jane White

Stephen Hancocks, OBE, Editor in Chief of the *British Dental Journal*

Phil Micans for his support and contribution to *Great Teeth For Life*

Foreword

Brian is one of life's enthusiasts. He is also one of life's dedicated carers. He cares passionately about his patients and, more particularly, about how dentistry, his chosen lifelong profession, can intervene to help patients in ways far beyond the traditional boundaries of dental treatment.

Over his years in dental practice in Buckinghamshire, he has come to develop an interest in holistic care for his patients, especially in the interplay between diet, general health, and the consequent effects on oral health. I suspect that history will show Brian to have been ahead of the game in this respect since there is currently much debate regarding the importance of including oral health as a part of general health, to the extent of a recent World Health Organization resolution urging that future preventive health programs link these two approaches.

As Brian writes here, "Diet, I believe, is vital for healthy bodies and teeth, and it is the core of this book," and his dedication to this shines through in page after page of heartfelt advice developed over years of daily practice, reading, attending lectures, and applying his personal convictions to the care of his patients.

Readers of this book will learn much about Brian's view of the interaction of diet and oral health, general health, and well-being and in doing so will help to disseminate his personal guiding philosophy: "If in doubt, don't."

Stephen Hancocks, OBE
Editor in Chief, *British Dental Journal*
September 2009

Introduction

Great Teeth for Life

Advice for My Readers

Before making decisions on changing lifestyle, diet, and/or starting a new supplement regime, research as much as possible. Read books and articles by well-respected experts. Use the Internet and follow references.

When you read articles in popular magazines and newspapers that appear to contradict common sense science—e.g., "Too much vitamin C is bad for you" and "Your amalgam fillings are completely safe"—ask these questions: "Can you show me the science?" and "Who funded the research and the scientists involved?" Even the Internet is full of misinformation, so beware!

My wish is that this book will provide information that, to a lesser or greater degree, will improve both the dental and general health and well-being of as many people as possible, especially the children of our world.

I believe that having the correct information is *power*:

Power to improve your health
Power to help others and to make choices that will benefit the planet and mankind

CHAPTER ONE

Why Should You Read This Book?

In my 1986 book, *The Natural Dentist*, I wrote the following:

> If, as a consequence of not washing our hands properly, they were to wither away, we should probably use soap and water rather more frequently than was entirely necessary. If our legs were to show a tendency to drop off when we ate the wrong foods, we would undoubtedly make sure that the right foods were totally predominant in our diet. Yet this is what is happening in our mouths: we are not eating a good diet, and thus the vast majority of us appear to be choosing to become dental cripples!
>
> Every day of my practicing career as a dentist, I observe some form of dental disease, either tooth decay or gum disease, and both of these, I believe, are almost totally preventable. And because they are so easily preventable, the frustration of dentists like myself can be readily appreciated. The most minor lifestyle changes—like better cleaning and a more sensible daily diet—can reduce disease in the mouth to almost negligible levels, yet somewhere along the line, the message has not gotten through, and it is still not getting through. Teeth are vital in so many ways—eating and good appearances are but two—but a majority seem not to care. A mere 50 percent of the population in the UK actually visits the dentist regularly, and dental care came only twentieth in surveys of spending priorities. In fact, it was not many years ago that it was accepted that you were lucky to still have your teeth after the age of twenty-one; often it's not a case of

saving for a house deposit or a car, but for a good set of false teeth!

This lemming-like attitude amazes and saddens me. When I—and indeed most dentists—tell patients how they can prevent dental disease, they often remark sarcastically: "Well, if I do everything you tell me to do, you're going to do yourself out of a job." It's touching, but somewhat ironic, that they should be worried about my well-being—my financial well-being in particular—to the detriment of their own health and that of their families. It could almost appear that they're trying, by ignoring their teeth, to keep dentists in business!

Two to three years later, the global worldwide prevalence of tooth decay and gum disease continues to grow unabated. With *Great Teeth for Life*, my sincerest wish is that my reader will use the information as a self-help manual.

Dental disease is preventable, resulting in less pain, less anxiety, less time and expense at the dentist, and improved health, not just in the mouth but throughout your body as well.

Nutrition is at the core of my book. "We are what we eat" is profoundly relevant. We are composed of what we consume: solids. To remain truly healthy in the twenty-first century is a challenge to us all. Holistic dentistry provides a way of meeting that challenge.

The inspiration for this latest book comes from thirty years of general practice as a holistic dental practitioner, during which time many patients have benefited from a preventative approach to dental health care. Regular attendance with our hygienists and me has meant that the concept of healthy teeth for life has become a reality for the majority of our patients, many now in their eighties and nineties. Those younger than sixteen have benefited the most, some before they were even born! It is heartwarming to see the vast majority of our teenage patients attend with good-looking, uncrowded teeth *and* zero fillings.

By seeing patients regularly, a holistic practitioner can often detect the early signs of disease. Even a simple greeting of "How are you?" has a diagnostic significance. When patients know and trust their practitioners, they will often disclose life stresses that, taken in the context of clinical findings, may well, for example, help in finding the causes of bleeding gums, tooth sensitivity, frequent mouth ulcers, or regular headaches.

By giving advice on healthy eating (not just avoiding sugars to prevent tooth decay) and giving up unhealthy habits such as smoking and excessive consumption of alcohol, improvements in dental health are accompanied by improved general health and well-being. Recently, many of my patients have been complaining of sensitive teeth, especially the younger generation. Regular consumption of fizzy drinks, even sparkling water, is often the cause. This leads to the thinning of the enamel of the teeth (acid erosion), making them sensitive to stimuli such as heat, cold, acidic and sweet foods, as well as touch, especially at the gum line of the teeth.

Regular attendance places a holistic practitioner in the unique position of being able to observe change in the patient's well-being. I believe in integrated holistic health—*body*, *mind*, and *spirit*. The holistic practitioner, of whatever specialization, looks at the individual as a whole person. Each part of the body is seen in relationship to the rest of the body, and any diagnosis is seen in terms of the body as a whole, and how treatment will benefit the patient physically, spiritually, and mentally. No part of the body is studied in isolation. By relating disease in the mouth to an imbalance in the body, the mouth becomes "a barometer of health." The holistic dentist can then also aspire to a much wider disease-prevention role in society. Beyond dental care, I endeavor to spend time with my patients, often guiding them to seek the advice of other holistic practitioners or suggesting relevant reading material.

There is no doubt that correct nutrition governs dental health. If nutrition and dentistry seem to be unlikely bedfellows, just consider the sugar question. The antipathy of dentists toward sugar in its more obvious confectionary forms is well known, and cutting out all sugar is a good first step toward improved dental health. The refined and processed foods so prevalent today are detrimental for physical and mental health, as well as dental health.

This was graphically illustrated by the research of an American dentist as long ago as the 1930s. Dr. Weston Price studied numerous isolated peoples who were still living on natural diets, far from the influences of Western civilization. Before they encountered modern foodstuffs such as white flours and sugars, they were healthy, happy, and dentally fit—with wide jaws, wide dental arches, and little tooth decay. Within a generation, however, the situation had drastically changed, and the younger, growing generation, without exception, had altered behaviorally and physically, displaying tooth decay, narrow dental arches and poor skeletal structures. *Nutrition and Physical Degeneration*, Dr. Price's book, is full of before and after pictures that provide spectacular confirmation that nutrition has everything to do with dental health of the teeth.[1]

Below is a clear example of how, within fifteen years, an Indian boy, having changed to a westernized diet, has terrible tooth decay. Other factors such as geography and environment have remained constant.[1]

---

1   Price, W., DDS. *Nutrition and Physical Degeneration, A Comparison of Primitive and Modern Diets and Their Effects.* La Mesa, CA: Price-Pottenger Nutrition Foundation, 1945, first published 1938

Great Teeth for Life

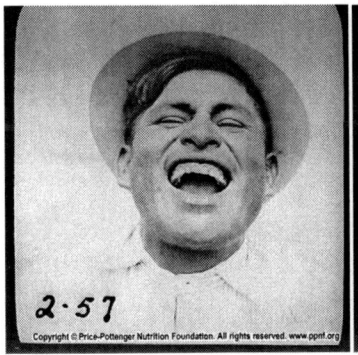 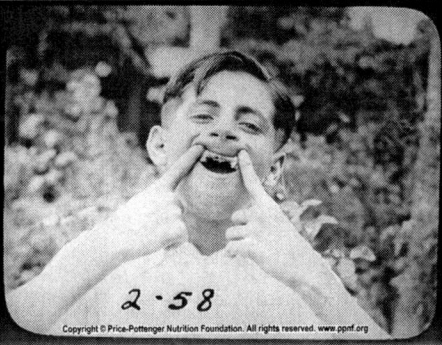

Fig 1 (a)
The Indian above lived on the coast of Peru, South America, where, like the ancestors of his tribe, he was living largely out of the sea, which provides an abundance of fish forms. His teeth are free from dental caries, and he has many physical characteristics that display the excellence of the nutrition of that group, both in his generation and in the hundreds of years preceding, as evidenced by burials.

Price Pottinger Nutrition Foundation

Fig 1 (b)
In contrast, we have a highly modernized Indian boy (above), also living on the coast in the port of Quayaquil, Ecuador. Dental caries have already robbed him in his boyhood of a large proportion of his teeth.

Both photographs were taken by Weston A. Price, DDS, and are copyrighted by the Price-Pottenger Nutrition Foundation and reproduced here with their permission.

Dr. Price has thousands of photographs showing similar before and after effects of the introduction of a civilized diet on isolated natives. This degenerative effect occurred regardless of whether the traditional diet was predominately meat, fish, mixed, or vegetarian.

Doctors and dentists are still largely overlooking the relationship between nutrition and health. Is this because most undergraduate medical training has only a small part of the curriculum devoted to nutrition? Using good nutrition as a means to good health seems to be a forgotten science.

An enormous number of phobias are built up around visiting the dentist, and certainly an image still persists of the dentist as "driller-filler." By making small lifestyle changes, visiting the dentist can be much less traumatic. By preventing the disease from developing, the treatment that is most feared will, in the majority of cases, simply not be required. I sincerely believe that *prevention* is the way forward if we want to create a healthy society, and we must start from before birth and continue throughout life.

The prevailing attitude is still to treat the disease, not the cause. As the world becomes more westernized, are we getting healthier? Considering heart disease, cancer, dementias, diabetes, allergies, arthritis, etc., I think not.

How much is spent on disease care? There is never enough. How much is spent on health care, i.e., prevention? Not enough. Is dental health any different from general health?

Do you know that most of the world's population today has some form of gum disease?

Do you also know how common tooth decay is today?

Even with all our technology, it is globally appalling. In 2007, a massive study of children's teeth in England, Scotland, and Wales was conducted.[2] These are the figures relating to those six years and under (an age when most children have not had the opportunity of receiving preventative advice from a dentist):

Children with tooth decay:

- England 38 percent
- Scotland 46 percent
- Wales 53 percent

Australia and the United States have recently reported similar figures. Globally, these statistics are not the exception but the norm! Just think of all these children, all over the world, condemned to perhaps a lifetime of dental disease, most of it preventable![3]

[2] The British Association for the Study of Community Dentistry (BASCD), results of 2005/2006 survey of five-year-olds within the NHS, release date 15 March 2007.

[3] Australia Tooth Decay—ABC News (Australia), 17 Dec 2007. Half of all six-year-olds have tooth decay. "A national children's dental

The Answer?

Holistic dentists believe that gum disease, ulcers, and other diseases of the soft tissues of the mouth are caused by poor nutrition. Gum disease is a case in point: if the body is poorly supplied nutritionally, then the mouth tissue will also suffer, for the blood that flows to the gums is the same blood that pumps through the heart and down to the toes. No part of the body can be viewed in isolation from the whole.

An example from the past: when sailors lacked fresh fruit and vegetables, they suffered from scurvy, which is a disease resulting from a shortage of vitamin C. The first signs of scurvy are swollen, bleeding gums! Dentists are in a unique position in our modern-day society. They have a wide knowledge of the disciplines of general medicine (although obviously not to the same degree as their medical colleagues), and they have a highly specialized knowledge of the mouth and its related disorders. They also see their patients on a regular basis, and thus are in a position to act as reviewers of health, operating a sort of early-warning system. A doctor may see a patient only when that patient is unwell and requires his services; a dentist will see patients at, ideally, six-month intervals and may be, as has often happened, the first one to spot the signs of early disease, a nutritional deficiency, or the inimitable symptoms of stress, of which the patient may not even be aware. Indeed, more than a few unexplained persistent headaches and backaches have been diagnosed and treated successfully by dentists investigating TMJ syndrome, a malfunction of the jaw alignment.

Screening for mouth cancer has now become an essential part of a regular checkup and dental examination. Early detection can save lives.

---

survey has shown the oral health of children from poorer families is declining."
U.S. Center for Disease Control and Prevention (CDC).
CDC Report April 2007: Tooth Decay: An Increasing Problem in Young Children."

Because the benefits of this medical-dental screening are potentially so important, dentists can widen their scope and play a more positive role in society's preventative health. If they succeed in reeducating the public dentally, they will be freer to concentrate on health counseling, advising on the growth and development of their new patients from as early as the preconceptual stage, and this can help to ensure the physical, medical, and dental health of the generations to come.

An analogy could be:

> *There was a dangerous bend in the road, where cars would crash over the cliff and into the gorge below.*
>
> *The "authorities" decided the best way to deal with this situation was to provide an efficient accident and emergency service to deal with the resulting casualties.*
>
> *Perhaps a better solution would have been to erect a safety barrier at the top of the cliff to prevent accidents before they happened. We can liken this to the provision of health care in most "civilized" countries, i.e., we have access to highly sophisticated health services to treat various diseases; however, we also need to erect the safety barrier to help us prevent diseases before they occur.*

My book is dedicated to holistic preventative health and to those who have suffered through ignorance and no fault of their own.

CHAPTER TWO

The Evolution of Dentistry: The Good, the Bad, and the Ugly

The history of dentistry is interlaced with archaeology, diet, inventiveness (sometimes magnificently creative, sometimes quite horrific), pain, social customs, and politics. And that history is long, for man, of course, has always had teeth, as well as, for the most part, tooth decay and gum disease. That we are still suffering from these same diseases centuries later, after all the advances in scientific knowledge, is amazing to me in my capacity as both a conventional and natural dentist: sugar, for instance, was recognized early as a cause of rotten teeth, but now we appear to be eating more of it than ever before. The fact that less than 50 percent of the population goes to the dentist regularly in the UK was highlighted recently: "New survey reveals shocking discrepancy between what parents spend on sweets and sugary drinks and their level of spending on their children's dental care ..." More than one thousand families across the UK took part in an online survey, and the results point to a growing neglect and lack of education in oral hygiene.[4]

In the Beginning

Teeth, made of one of the hardest natural substances, and certainly the most indestructible part of the human body, have proved vital clues in the search for our past. From skulls found in prehistoric sites around the world, and dating from many periods, the development of "modern" man can be traced. As man evolved over hundreds of thousands of years, his physical appearance slowly altered. The most important change was in the shape of his skull as the size of his brain increased; the second most important was in the shape

---

4   *The Probe*, April 2009, Vol. 51, No. 4.

of his jaw and in the size and variety of his teeth. The latter, from present-day dental examinations, seem to have suffered little from tooth decay and gum disease.

Early ancestors of man had formidable canines, or eyeteeth, like today's baboons, but *Homo habilis*, or "handy man," who lived about 1.75 million years ago, had canines that were as small as our own today. The canines were fighting teeth, with which to threaten, pierce, puncture, and tear. Think of the baboon's most aggressive gesture: throwing back the head and opening the mouth to display the teeth. The decrease in size of those canines in man probably went hand in hand with his development of the use of weapons and tools; now he was no longer reliant on physical attributes such as claws or teeth, but could make and design his own. Thus the necessity for those canines declined (although Dracula still makes a basically primitive use of his!), and this newfound ability, so amply demonstrated in teeth, was probably the key by which man ultimately gained mastery over all other species.

As brain size altered, so did the shape of the jaw. The brain size of *Australopithecus*, who lived in Africa some five million years ago, was little larger than his ape cousin, and his jaws were prominent, with large and powerful teeth, in order to chew tough grains and raw meat. By the time of *Homo erectus*, who lived 4.5 million years later, the brain had enlarged and the jaw had decreased in size, as had the teeth. *Homo erectus* used fire for warmth and probably for cooking too. As cooked meat is easier to chew than raw, the large flat molar or back teeth that earlier forms of man had developed were not as necessary. Those enormous teeth and massive jaws could thus be reduced in size to the more refined physical characteristics of modern man, and these have finally evolved over the last thirty thousand years.

If toolmaking was the key to man's dominance over the rest of the animal world, and the cooking of food heralded the beginnings of modern man, cooking food could also be said, perhaps, to mark the beginnings of dental disease. A good diet is vital for healthy bodies and teeth, and it is the core of this book. In a world entirely free of all our modern pollutants, primitive man lived a healthy—if

Great Teeth for Life

relatively short and dangerous—life, eating a healthy diet of raw nuts, seeds, grasses, and raw meats and fish.

As a consequence of this diet, the dental arches in both upper and lower jaws were broad to allow room for the biting incisors and canines, as well as the grinding molars at the back. Foods that require active chewing were, and are, good for the jaws and teeth. This spaciousness of the arch is still the prime requisite of a good jaw and healthy teeth today, and our smaller jaws have to rely on orthodontics, which may necessitate the removal of teeth to prevent crowding, and thus the places between the teeth are where the disease-carrying bacteria can flourish.

So, as man began to cook his food—together with processing it (for the processing of grains into flour, for example, was also an early practice)—jaws decreased in size, teeth became more crowded, and mouth disease began.[5]

The quality of this early food would have been much better, in terms of an organic environment with a correct balance of vitamins and minerals, so the proportion of disease would have been small. There were undeniably other factors in promoting tooth decay. The teeth of some Bronze Age skulls show decay, which is probably the result of grinding on pieces of bone, shell, or grit, which inevitably wore down the surface of the teeth, creating holes into which bacteria could enter. However, if we were able to compare, say, one hundred primitive men with a similar number of present-day men, the teeth of the former would undoubtedly be in much better condition, despite the complete absence of dentists, toothbrushes, and toothpaste!

---

5 (a) Hillson, S. *Teeth*, 2nd Edition, Series Cambridge Manuals in Archaeology, Cambridge University Press.
(b) Neely, A.; Holford, L.; Loe, T.; Aneurad, H.; Boysen, A. "The Natural History of Periodontal Disease in Humans: Risk Factors for Tooth Loss in Caries-Free Subjects Receiving No Oral Health Care." J Clin Periodontol, 2005;32, (9): 984–993, Denmark: Blackwell Publishing Ltd.

Brian Halvorsen, BDS, LDS RCS

Dentistry in Antiquity

There were no Stone Age dentists because, overall, the teeth of Stone Age man were in good condition. But shortly afterward, at least in terms of the history of man, ancient texts from all over the world begin to record diseases of the teeth and how to treat them. A Sumerian clay tablet, "The Legend of the Worm," dating from around 5000 BC, gives advice on how to rid the teeth of the small worms believed to cause toothache. This tooth-eating worm theory was to be associated with tooth decay for many centuries thereafter, and it is not so fanciful when we consider that many of the bacteria that cause decay are literally worm shaped. Over one thousand years later, a Sanskrit text had details on surgery, and in the famous medical "Ebers Papyrus," discovered in Egypt around 1862 and written in about 1500 BC (but copied, it is thought, from earlier papyri), many ideas of treatment are listed, although no mention is made of any surgical or restorative procedures.[6]

Indeed, from the thousands of mummies examined over the years, the ancient Egyptians, those of the upper classes anyway, appeared to have suffered greatly from dental disease. Jawbones and teeth show evidence of rampant gum disease and tooth decay, and the resultant infection of bone known as "osteomyelitis." Although it is commonly believed that ancient Egypt enjoyed the services of experts on teeth, who made dental appliances and fillings from gold, no proof of any dentistry has been found in any mummies. But if these dentists had existed, their "work" would have been evident in the mouths of those entombed as mummies, and if they were rich and important enough to face the afterlife, they would certainly have sought relief from their pain in the *here and now*.

It was not until the time of the Etruscans, a people who lived in what is now Tuscany in Italy, and whose civilization stretched roughly from the eighth to the fourth centuries BC, that we have evidence of a high level of dentistry. Partial dentures and early dental bridges have been found in tombs: bands of gold hold together the natural and artificial or substitute teeth (one such found was the tooth of

---

6   Lindsay, L. *A Short History of Dentistry*. John Bale, Sons & Danielsson, Ltd. 1933, pp 8–9.

Great Teeth for Life

a calf). No attempt was made to hide these golden bands, which covered a large proportion of the crown of the teeth, thus suggesting that they were worn with pride rather than in shame, a little like the gold teeth flashing proudly from many Mediterranean and African mouths today.

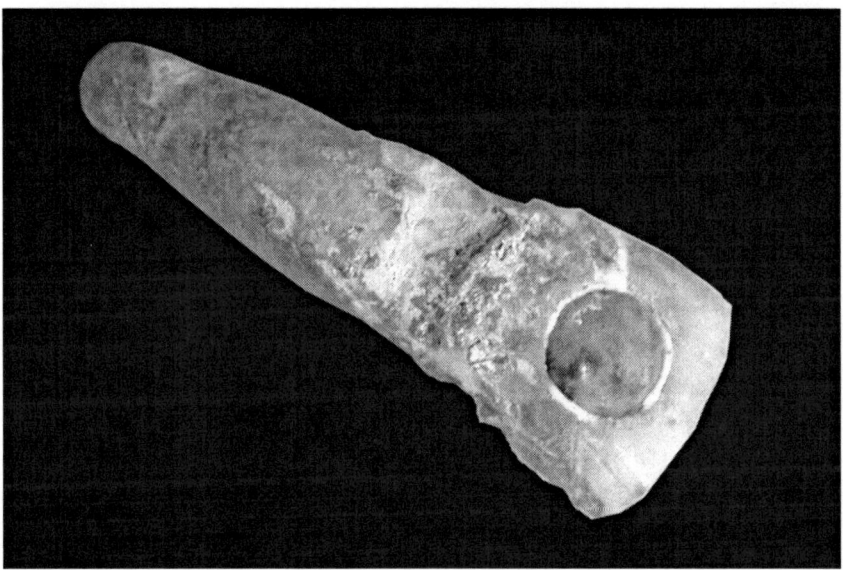

Fig. 2
Precious Stone Inlay in a Front Tooth circa 1000 AD
An example of Mayan cosmetic dentistry, showing great skill with primitive tools

British Dental Association
Ref. 7688c
Credit: Photograph by Fil Gierlinski, reproduced courtesy of the British Dental Association Museum

The ancient Greeks and Romans suffered from tooth decay and gum disease as well. Hippocrates, the Greek "Father of Medicine," recommended extraction when teeth were decayed or loose, although later writers, like Aristotle, were better dental anatomists. Roman medical writer Aulus Cornelius Celsus wrote, in about 25 BC to AD 35, of dental matters very near to the heart of this book: that poor teeth result from the processed foods of civilization. In his De Re Medicina, he advised the inhabitants of towns and cities to wash their mouths out well daily to prevent tooth decay; peasants did not need to bother, apparently, because of their simple and unrefined diet. Caius Plinius Secundus, or "Pliny the Elder" (AD 23-79),[7] echoed some of Celsus's ideas: "A man's breath becomes infected by the bad quality of the food, by the bad state of his teeth, and still more by old age." This apparent scientific modernity is somewhat dashed by his renowned inability to distinguish between fact and fiction: he recorded a current belief that a frog tied to the jaws would make loose teeth firm![8]

In antiquity, then, there was a variable degree of dental sophistication, but an unvarying amount of dental disease. It is difficult to generalize, of course, because the current evidence relates primarily to a particular social class, upper classes who were buried in a more durable manner or whose ills were treated and recorded by their physicians. It does seem, however, that dentistry went hand in hand with civilization as with any advancement of science, and as exhibited by the dental silence of the Dark Ages of the barbarians following the collapse of the Roman Empire. With civilization came a "civilized" and thus refined diet; and with that came the diseases associated with diet, primarily tooth decay and gum disease.

Dentistry in the Middle Ages

The Chinese used acupuncture to alleviate toothache as early as 2700 BC, and the Arabians kept dental skills and research alive. Abulcasis (1050–1122) was regarded as the greatest Arabian surgeon of the Middle Ages, and his *De Chirurgia* remained a standard medical textbook for centuries thereafter. He set broken jaws with wire splints, improved extraction instruments, treated harelips successfully, and was perhaps the first dental hygienist; in his book, he illustrated many different dental scalers and described in detail the process of scaling, which is the scraping of tartar, or calculus, from the teeth.

---

7   Pliny. *Natural History*, A Selection, translated by John F. Healy, Penguin Classics, 1991.
8   Woodforde, J. *The Strange Story of False Teeth*, London: Routledge & Kegan Paul, 1968, 12.

In Britain, it was not until 1308 that some semblance of organization attached itself to those who extracted teeth. The barber-surgeons formed themselves into a guild, and they were divided into two groups, including those who practiced barberry proper: phlebotomy, or bloodletting, and tooth extraction. This is the meaning behind the colors of the traditional barber's pole, red for blood and white for teeth. The second group practiced general surgery. The guild remained active until 1745, after which the barbers separated to form a guild of their own.[9]

In Europe, Guy de Chauliac (1309–1386), a French surgeon, wrote extensively on the teeth, although reiterating much of what Abulcasis had written 250 years earlier. He used soporific drugs to subdue pain, and in some manuscript copies of his great treatise, *Chirurgia Magna*, there appears for the first time the word "dentista."[10] A century later, Giovanni Vigo, an Italian surgeon, advocated careful excavating and shaping of a tooth cavity before filling with gold leaf. Amboise Pare, a French surgeon, recorded transplantation of teeth and claimed that dental decay was caused by worms (a belief continuing into the late sixteenth century),[11] and stated that preventative measures such as filing the teeth, removing tartar, and general mouth hygiene should be undertaken.

For many years in Britain, only the barber-surgeons and their extraction methods were available, besides those of their main rivals, against whom the guild bitterly railed: the itinerant and unqualified tooth-drawers. These gentlemen, often wearing necklaces of teeth or hats decorated with teeth, would frequent markets and fairs, offering their services. Drums were beaten loudly and music played to drown the screams of the unfortunate sufferers. That they were many, and

9 Prinz, H. *Dental Chronology: A record of the more important historic events in the evolution of Dentistry*. London: Henry Kimpton, 1945, 35.
See Also: Lindsay, L. *A Short History of Dentistry*. John Bale, Sons & Danielsson, Ltd. 1933, 8–9.
And Hoffmann-Axthelm, W. *History of Dentistry*, Quintessence Publishing, 1981.
10 Prinz, H. *Dental Chronology: A record of the more important historic events in the evolution of Dentistry*. London: Henry Kimpton, 1945, 35.
11 Prinz, H. *Dental Chronology: A record of the more important historic events in the evolution of Dentistry*. London: Henry Kimpton, 1945, 38.

that their services were needed as well as dreaded, is evidenced by the prolific paintings and prints over the years of the common people suffering their attentions. The main instruments used were pliers or forceps, pelicans (with a claw to pry a tooth out), and elevators, which had a tapering blade to elevate the roots of bad teeth.

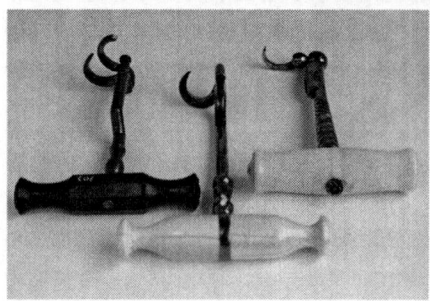

Fig. 3 (a)
Teeth extraction instruments used between the eighteenth and nineteenth century

*British Dental Association
Ref. BDA Col. 45
Credit:
Photograph by Fil Gierlinski, reproduced courtesy of the British Dental Association Museum*

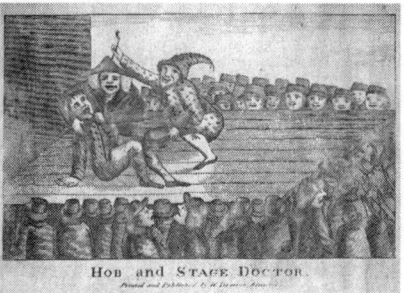

Fig. 3 (b)
Tooth pulling as entertainment, sixteenth century—remember, *no numbing!*

*British Dental Association
Ref. 10428
Credit:
Photograph by Fil Gierlinski, reproduced courtesy of the British Dental Association Museum*

The horrors of dental pain and tooth extraction are perhaps most clearly exemplified by the Virgin Queen Elizabeth I. She suffered severely with toothache from her childhood onward and, according to a German visitor to her court, had black teeth, which he said was characteristic of the English in general because of their great love of sugar and sweetmeats, sweet puddings, cakes, candied fruits, etc., which are still the most famed aspect of English cuisine even today. It is recorded that Elizabeth, when once suffering badly from toothache, could only be persuaded to have the tooth out by Bishop Aylmer, who volunteered to have one of his drawn first to show that the pain wasn't as bad as she might expect. Greater love hath no man.

Great Teeth for Life

False teeth in England were rare at this time, and to fill out a mouth bereft of teeth, Queen Elizabeth I would pad her jaws and cheeks with cloths in the interest of vanity.[12] Many of her portraits, and indeed those of many other well-to-do people of the period, do show that teeth were few, if not completely lacking. It is a particularly interesting exercise for dentists and dental students, but if you go to a gallery or a historic house, look at the jaw position in portraits and note how near the nose is to the chin. Many people in the portraits were obviously young and lacked teeth, and this is probably why none of the sitters are smiling or showing teeth! Until the end of the seventeenth century in Britain, dental progress was negligible. There were attempts, though, at dentures for those who lacked teeth.[13] Robert Herrick (1591–1674), a Cavalier poet responsible for the immortal line "Gather ye rosebuds while ye may," wrote an ode called "Upon Glasco":

> *Glasco had none, but now some teeth has got;*
> *Which though they furre, will neither ake nor rot.*
> *Six teeth he has, whereof twice two are known*
> *Made of a haft that was a mutton bone*
> *Which not for use, but meerly for the sight,*
> *He wears all day and drawes those teeth at night.*

These dentures, often made from animal bone or carved from ivory for the very rich, conjure up a picture of a toothless nation, particularly the upper classes, who would be unable to eat or speak properly. More sophisticated dentures with which their wearer could eat or speak without clicking, movement, or displacement—even shooting out—were not available until at least the beginning of the eighteenth century.

In 1683 a Dutchman, Antony van Leeuwenhoek, described for the first time the presence of tiny animals in the debris around the human teeth, and he opined that their numbers in one mouth

---

12   Woodforde, J. *The Strange Story of False Teeth*, London: Routledge & Kegan Paul, 1968, 19–20.

13   Woodforde, J. *The Strange Story of False Teeth*, London: Routledge & Kegan Paul, 1968, 23.

probably exceeded the number of men in the country. He had taken some bacterial plaque from his own mouth, and he was the first person to look at it under a microscope.[14] In 1700, the French College of Surgeons inaugurated a dental department and created the first examinations for dental practitioners. In 1712, one Nicol Facussi successfully implanted teeth obtained from corpses, and the practice of transplantation was to continue and expand over the next couple of centuries. Even one hundred years later, after the Battle of Waterloo, hordes of scavengers raided the corpses of soldiers lying on the battlefield to extract their teeth for use in dentures.[15]

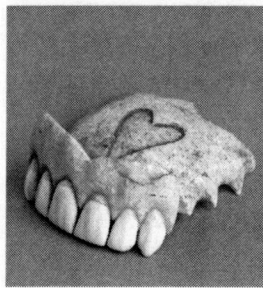 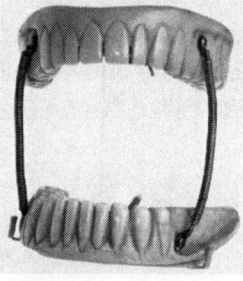 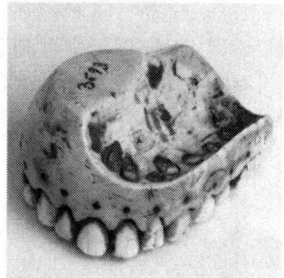

Fig. 4 (a)
Carved ivory denture given as romantic gift. Circa 1790.

British Dental Association
Ref. BDA Col. 18
Credit:
Photograph by Fil Gierlinski, reproduced courtesy of the British Dental Association Museum

Fig. 4 (b)
Carved ivory denture with piano wire springs. Circa 1790.

British Dental Association
Ref. BDA Col. 11
Credit:
Photograph by Fil Gierlinski, reproduced courtesy of the British Dental Association Museum

Fig. 4 (c)
The denture of Sir Edmund Burke (1729–1797). Human teeth, ivory base. Sir Edmund was a renowned Parliamentarian and speaker—imagine trying to speak eloquently with this in your mouth!

British Dental Association
Ref. BDA Col. 16
Credit:
Photograph by Fil Gierlinski, reproduced courtesy of the British Dental Association Museum

---

14 Prinz, H. *Dental Chronology: A record of the more important historic events in the evolution of Dentistry*. London: Henry Kimpton, 1945, 57.
15 Woodforde, J. *The Strange Story of False Teeth*, London: Routledge & Kegan Paul, 1968, 62.

The Beginnings of Modern Dentistry

In 1728, Pierre Fauchard (1678–1761), a French surgeon-dentist, published two volumes that made dental history. They were the first systematic attempt to record a complete picture of the practice of dentistry, and they brought about a distinction and separation of the practices of dentistry and surgery. From that point forward, the science itself, as well as treatment, prosthesis (the replacement by artificial limbs or teeth), and the making of dentures, crowns, and bridges, became more sophisticated.[16]

In 1746, Pierre Mouton described the making of the gold shell crown for the first time. In 1757, the theory of worms in the teeth was disproved; in 1790, John Greenwood, an American dentist, invented a dental foot drill (he was also one of George Washington's dentists and made him several sets of teeth); and in 1771, John Hunter, FRS, a surgeon and pathologist, published *The Natural History of the Human Teeth*, which formed the basis for all modern texts on the jaw and teeth. He also experimented with the transplanting of sound teeth. This barbaric practice became quite popular, and newspapers carried advertisements asking for natural human teeth. Poor unfortunates with good sound teeth, mainly children, would have them wrenched painfully from their mouths, and these freshly extracted teeth would then promptly be implanted into the mouths of wealthy recipients. For this, the donor could be paid two guineas (a large amount then). Suitable slaves would also be used as donors, and they of course would be paid a cheaper rate.[17]

---

16   Prinz, H. *Dental Chronology: A record of the more important historic events in the evolution of Dentistry.* London: Henry Kimpton, 1945, 61.

17   Prinz, H. *Dental Chronology: A record of the more important historic events in the evolution of Dentistry.* London: Henry Kimpton, 1945. And Woodforde, J. *The Strange Story of False Teeth*, London: Routledge & Kegan Paul, 1968, 84.

Brian Halvorsen, BDS, LDS RCS

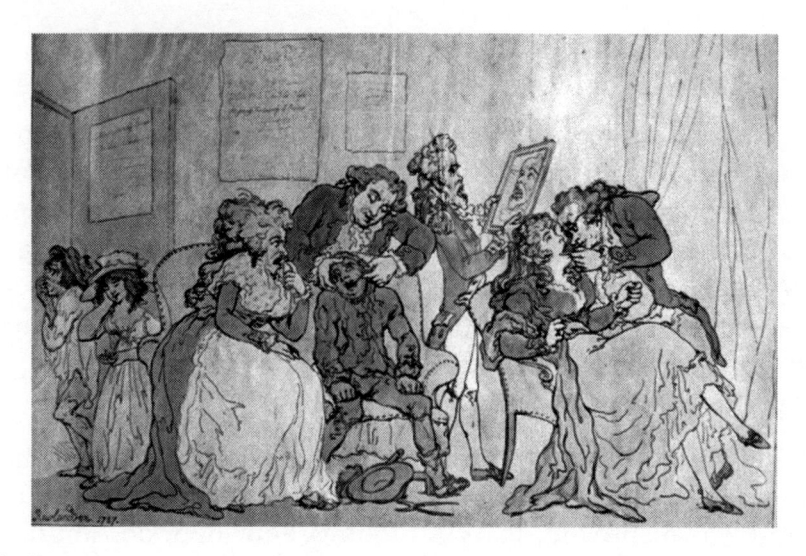

Fig. 5
Transplanting of teeth. Illustration by Thomas Rowlandson (Remember, no anesthetic!)
British Dental Association Ref. 7713
Credit: Photograph by Fil Gierlinski, reproduced courtesy of the British Dental Association Museum

And in 1775, Paul Revere, subject of Longfellow's poem "Paul Revere's Ride," was perhaps the first dentist to be called upon to identify a corpse, killed at the battle of Bunker Hill, from its dental work.[18]

At the beginning of the nineteenth century, Joseph Fox was the first dental surgeon to be appointed to Guy's Hospital in London. By this time, tooth filling had become more common, and he was advocating a mixture of bismuth, lead, and tin. This was presumably as dangerous as the mercury that began to be used a few years later, cropping up again in 1826 when a French dentist used a filling amalgam of filings from silver five-franc pieces mixed with mercury. When, in 1833, the Crawcour brothers introduced a similar amalgam to America, their methods were the cause of the "amalgam war"[19] of about 1835–1850, when the American Dental

---

18 Prinz, H. *Dental Chronology: A record of the more important historic events in the evolution of Dentistry.* London: Henry Kimpton, 1945, 73.

19 Prinz, H. *Dental Chronology: A record of the more important historic events in the evolution of Dentistry.* London: Henry Kimpton, 1945, 96.

Association rescinded the statement that the use of amalgam was declared to be malpractice.

In 1844, Horace Wells, a Connecticut dentist, demonstrated the anesthetic properties for dentistry of laughing gas (nitrous oxide), and thereafter a new era in tooth extraction began. In the same year, plaster of Paris was introduced for taking impressions of the teeth, another leap forward for those who had to wear ill-fitting dentures (measured up until then with compasses and, if they were lucky, wax). A few years later, Edwin Truman,[20] Queen Victoria's dentist, introduced gutta-percha, a latex gum derived from Malaysian trees, as the basis for artificial dentures, and he also coated the Atlantic cable with gutta-percha, thus protecting it from the corrosion of seawater. It was also used in golf balls and chewing gum! In 1848, Thomas Evans of Paris used vulcanite (a hard material made by heating rubber with sulphur) as a base for artificial dentures. He made one such denture for Charles Goodyear Sr. in 1854. A few years later, Charles Goodyear Jr. patented the use of caoutchouc, or rubber, as a base for artificial dentures, and the Goodyear Dental Vulcanite Company received thereafter a royalty on every denture sold![21]

In 1891, the "grand old man in dentistry," Green Vardiman Black (1836–1915) of Chicago, began the process of preventative dentistry proper. He standardized cavity preparation—dentists still know Black's cavity classification today, and his research revolutionized the use of amalgam fillings.[22] With the dawning of the twentieth century, medicine and dentistry entered a new era following the development of significant scientific discoveries. Over one hundred years have elapsed since one of the first films, that of a jaw and teeth, was developed from the use of X-rays. At about the same time, the first local anesthetics were being used, an extremely potent mixture of cocaine and morphine. Today's dentists would

---

20 Prinz, H. *Dental Chronology: A record of the more important historic events in the evolution of Dentistry.* London: Henry Kimpton, 1945, 102.
21 Hoffmann-Axthelm, W. *History of Dentistry,* Quintessence Publishing, 1981.
22 Hoffmann-Axthelm, W. *History of Dentistry*, Quintessence Publishing, 1981.

certainly recognize equipment and techniques used in the latter part of the nineteenth century.

During the Boer War (1899–1902),[23] poor dental health nearly cost the British their eventual victory. Unlike today, the British Army had a medical Core but no dental division. The average soldier had very poor dental health, a dental infection often leading to a serious illness and making him unfit to fight. When dentists were eventually sent to South Africa to attend to the troops, the only treatment was extractions, leaving the soldiers unable to chew their tough food rations! More troops were unable to fight in the Boer War due to their dental condition than were actually killed.[24]

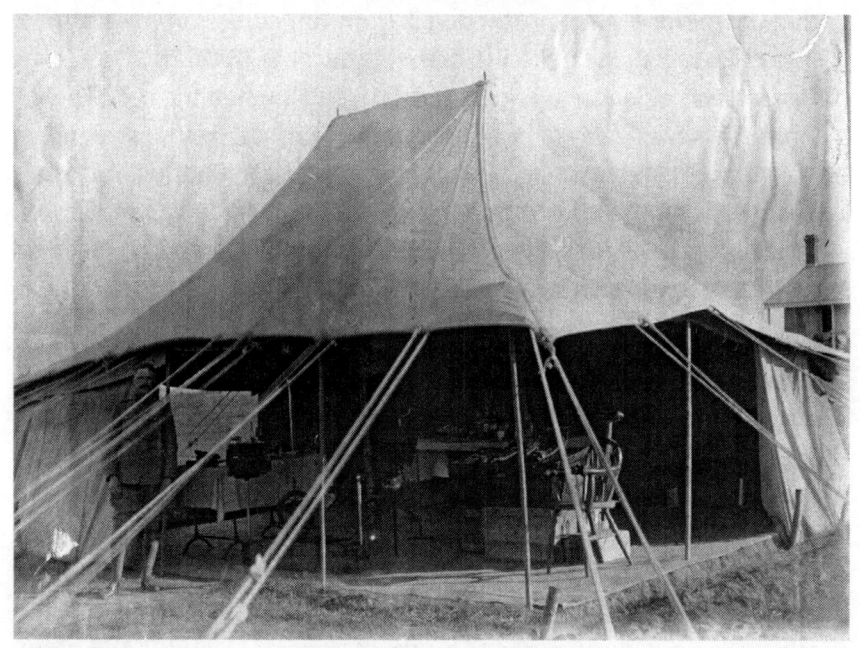

Fig. 6
E. W. Corfe (Surgeon) outside his tent during the Boer War.
British Dental Association Ref. A9
Credit: *Photograph by Fil Gierlinski, reproduced courtesy of the British Dental Association Museum*

23 Ward VH. *Ex Dentibus Ensis: A History of the Army Dental Service*; RADC Historical Museum, 1997.
24 Pain, S. "Can't Bite, Can't Fight." New Scientist, 10 March 2007, http://www.newscientist.com/article/mg19325942.200-cant-bite-cant-fight.html

The term "trench mouth" derived from World War I. A combination of poor nutrition, poor oral hygiene, and extreme stress led to a condition called acute ulcerative gingivitis. This and other incapacitating dental diseases led to the formation of the Royal Army Dental Corps.

It's interesting that the conditions in the trenches, leading to severe and rapidly spreading gum disease, is only a more obvious etiology of the causes of gum disease today!

Dentistry As a Profession

In the seventeenth and eighteenth centuries, there was no real profession of dentistry, but as science improved, there was a divide. Some dentists became very skilful, studying anatomy of jaws and teeth, performing skilful operations, and using sophisticated instruments. There were also those who were unskilled and unqualified; these "dentists" got their work through advertising at fairgrounds, etc.

In 1839, the birth of organized dentistry occurred, with the foundation of the first dental school in Baltimore, Maryland, in the United States; the first dental magazine (*American Journal of Dental Science*); and the first dental society (American Society of Dental Science). In England, it was not until 1878 that the Dentists Act of that year gave the General Medical Council the power to examine and register suitably qualified dentists.[25] However, it did not outlaw unqualified dentists, and you could still pull teeth without any qualification at all. In 1880, with the founding of the British Dental Association, dentistry became a profession in Britain, but it was not until 1921 that unregistered dentists were outlawed. There may be people alive today who had much of their early dental experiences at the hands of totally unqualified persons![26]

---

25   Lindsay, L. *A Short History of Dentistry*. John Bale, Sons & Danielsson, Ltd. 1933, 84.

26   Prinz, H. *Dental Chronology; A record of the more important historic events in the evolution of Dentistry*. London: Henry Kimpton, 1945, 96.

Brian Halvorsen, BDS, LDS RCS

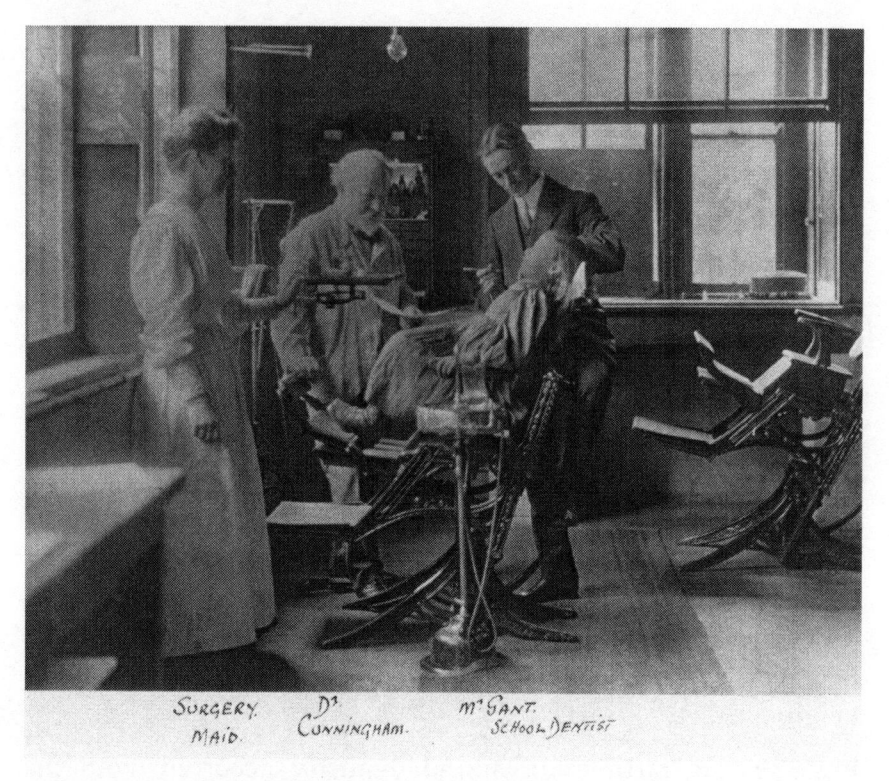

Fig. 7
George Cunningham, founder of the Cambridge Dental Institute for Children, one of the first established in the UK, in 1907.
British Dental Association Ref. A75
Credit: Photograph by Fil Gierlinski, reproduced courtesy of the British Dental Association Museum

In the early part of the twentieth century, most dentistry was carried out in private practices, although there were some dental hospitals in large cities. Dental disease was prevalent, and for the vast majority of the population, extraction was the only treatment for the relief of pain. In England, before the National Health Service, dentures were extremely expensive, and many people had to go without, as old newsreel cuttings of the thirties and forties amply illustrate. Indeed, it is not so long since a full set of dentures was a prized twenty-first birthday present; today it might be a mini car! The nervous middle-aged patient of today often remembers bad experiences of the past—memories of

Great Teeth for Life

austere waiting rooms and antiseptic-smelling surgeries mingled with visions of bloody spittoons and treadle drills.

With dental disease so widespread, the dentist could easily become hardened to pain and suffering. The priorities were to remove as much infection from the mouth as possible because, before the use of effective antibiotics, dental infections could be life threatening. There were undoubtedly dentists who exhibited a caring and preventative approach, but the image created in the populace was one of fear.

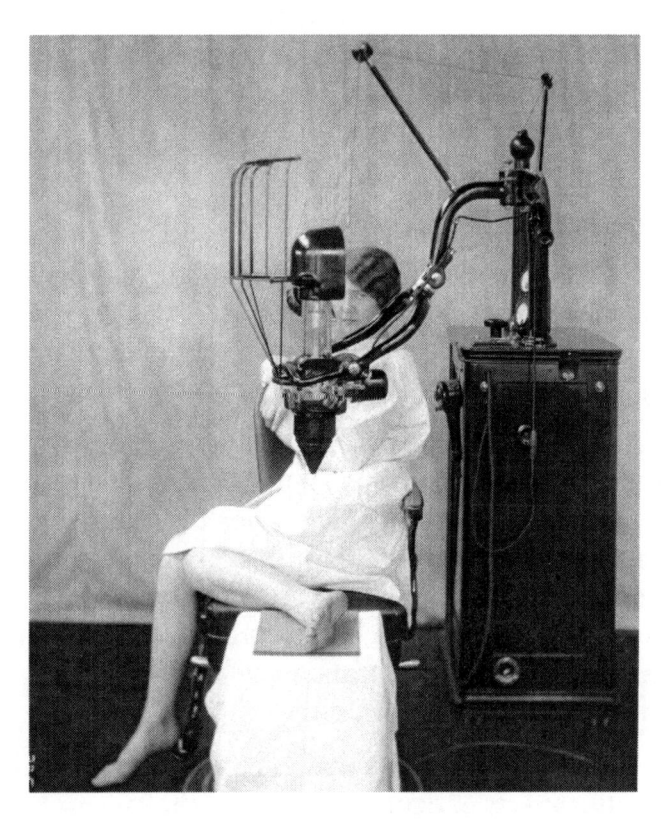

Fig. 8
Advert for an X-ray machine! Ritter (USA)—The first X-ray machine in 1920. Dentists in those days needed glamour models in order to be persuaded to buy dental equipment!
British Dental Association Ref. 10309
Credit: Photograph by Fil Gierlinski, reproduced courtesy of the British Dental Association Museum

Since the 1950s, the emphasis on dentistry in modern societies has evolved from extraction and dentures to conservative dentistry and, in the last thirty years, to education and prevention.

Conservative Dentistry

Advances in dental technology—such as high-speed drills, dental materials, and techniques—can provide the patient with crowns, bridges, implants, and root fillings. In fact, a means to have, fixed in the jaw, teeth for life. Today's dentistry can be provided pain free and safe from infection in comfortable surgeries, a far cry from the fairground tooth puller who had an assistant beat a loud drum to muffle the screams of his victims!

Education and Prevention

Since the 1970s, dental hygienists, therapists, and dental health educators have been trained to provide valuable preventative services, especially for patients who attend dental practices regularly. Just like a car, regular maintenance is essential.

Regular attendance to dentists and their teams has played a major role in reducing dental disease, i.e., tooth decay and gum disease. In most developed countries, dental health is slowly improving. Recent surveys have shown that this improvement in dental health appears to be confined to certain socioeconomic groups.[27] Toothbrush and toothpaste manufacture has contributed to this improvement through the education and awareness given via their extensive marketing and advertising.

Let us not lose sight of the fact that dentistry through the ages has addressed the effects of dental disease, not the causes. Today is no different; we now have very good rescue services at the bottom of the cliff, but we do little to provide the fence at the top of the cliff. Good and correct nutrition from before birth and throughout life is genuine holistic prevention!

---

27 "Tooth Decay; An Increasing Problem in Young Children." April 2007, U.S. Center for Disease Control and Prevention (CDC) report.

CHAPTER THREE

Teeth and Jaws: Get to Know This Vital Part of Your Body

The formation of teeth and jaws is a top priority in nature's order of things. Astonishingly, the milk, or baby, teeth are already beginning to calcify, or harden, in the jaw of the embryo as early as ten weeks after conception, probably just when the pregnancy is being confirmed. Teeth are a priority because primitive man could not have survived without them, as he would not have been able to eat. Even in times of severe hardship or malnutrition, a baby will develop teeth. The bones of a starving child might show gross skeletal problems such as rickets, but the teeth, although they will probably be affected (by what dentally we call "hypo," or "under," calcification), will still be present and be in fairly adequate shape. The bones might be so affected that a child could not walk, but in terms of nature's priorities, our early ancestors would have died if they could not have chewed their raw food.

Teeth and jaws, therefore, are a vital consideration right from the start of life, and I shall cover these both here and in the next chapter. I would first like to describe the basic structures of teeth and jaws, and some factors that can affect their initial formation.

The Teeth

People start off with twenty milk, or baby, teeth—the deciduous teeth (dentally, "deciduous" means exactly the same as it does botanically: deciduous teeth are shed like the leaves from a tree). Thereafter, we are the proud possessors of thirty-two permanent teeth. The variety of these teeth, at both stages of tooth development, shows clearly that man is an omnivore, that he does not have a specialization for eating either grass or meat.

The incisors, or front teeth, are for cutting; the pointed canines are for tearing, revealing a meat-eating ancestry (like dogs and the big cats); and the molars at the back are the flat grinding teeth to cope with the chewing of tough raw meats, grasses, and grains. Overall, we have good jaws and sets of teeth to cope with most types of food.

To define the teeth more clearly, it is easiest to use the approach of the dentist, in that dental language is a sort of scientific shorthand. Which could help you understand a little more of what is going on the next time you go to the dentist!

The dentist divides the mouth up into quadrants, with each side possessing a matching number of teeth—five deciduous and eight permanent. By specifying, say, the upper-left quadrant, this means left from the patient's point of view, not his own. In the United Kingdom, teeth are numbered from one to eight, using the front tooth as one and the wisdom tooth as eight. Each quadrant of the mouth can then be described. Because the teeth are only duplicated on each side, there aren't any variations unless a tooth is missing. Basically, no quadrant is different from another, which immediately simplifies an understanding of the language of the mouth.

In further defining a tooth, six more points must be considered:

1. Is it a deciduous or permanent tooth?
2. Is it an incisor (1 or 2), a canine (3), a pre-molar (4 or 5), or a molar (6, 7, or 8)?
3. Is it maxillary (upper jaw) or mandibular (lower jaw)?
4. If it is an incisor, is it a central incisor (1) or a lateral incisor (2)?
5. If it is a premolar, is it a first (number 4, that nearest the front of the mouth) or second (5, the next one back)?
6. If it is a molar, is it a first (6), second (7), or third (8)?

Many of these particular questions depend, of course, on the age of the owner of the teeth. The first molars grow at around six years old; the second appear at about twelve; and the third, the wisdom teeth, appear usually in the late teens, or early twenties.

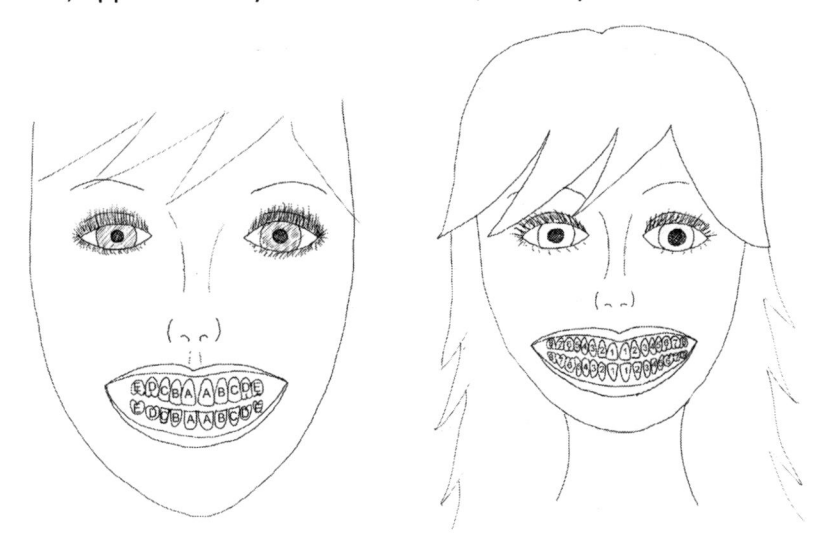

Fig. 9 (a)
Deciduous (Baby) Teeth

Fig. 9 (b)
Permanent (Adult) Teeth

Illustrations by Caroline White, copyright Brian Halvorsen 2010

In the deciduous dentition, the terminology is slightly different. Although divided similarly into quadrants, the teeth are defined as A, B, C, D, and E instead of one through eight. A baby has a central incisor (A), a lateral incisor (B), a canine (C), a first molar (D), and a second molar (E). Charts for the dates of eruption of both deciduous and permanent teeth are shown in chapter 3.

The Structure of a Tooth

Each tooth has five additional aspects: its surfaces. This is how they are defined dentally: the top or biting surface is the occlusal; the side nearest the cheeks is the buccal; the side nearest the tongue is the lingual; the mesial is the surface nearest to the front of the mouth; and the distal is the surface farthest away from the front of the mouth. It will help when brushing your teeth to remember the five surfaces, which must be cleaned regularly!

Each tooth is rooted into the gums and held firmly in place by the jawbone. In a healthy tooth, there is no direct contact between root and bone; between them there is a layer of what we call periodontal fibers or ligaments that hold the teeth in the bone like little hammocks. You can test this yourself by moving one of your hopefully healthy teeth from side to side. Instead of the tooth being rigid, it will move a tiny bit—not because the bone is soft, but because of these fibers. The reason for this is that when chewing, we need a little "give"; otherwise chewing could be as unpleasant as riding on a bumpy road in a car with no suspension.

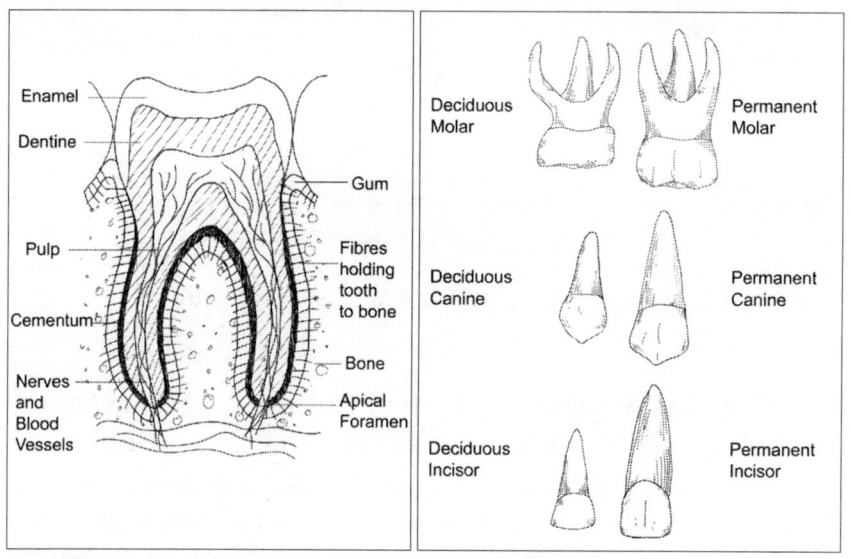

Fig. 10 (a)
Structure of a Molar Tooth

Fig. 10 (b)
Types of Teeth

Illustrations by Caroline White, copyright Brian Halvorsen, 2010

The root of the tooth is often much larger than the crown and, depending on what tooth it is, has one, two, or three roots. Occasionally, there are exceptions in the number and size. The root has canals flowing through it from the bone into the interior of the tooth. These contain blood vessels and nerve endings, and the little "hole" where they join the bone proper is called the apical foramen. This hole is important because of its functions and because its size can be constricted, especially with age, when you can get a generalized hardening and ageing of body tissue such as bone, arteries, and teeth. As far as teeth are concerned, though, this is not necessarily a bad thing, for if there were to be a cutting off of the nerve supply to the interior pulp of the tooth, all the painful trials that can accompany the nerve endings of teeth are brought to an end (although the tooth will now suffer the tribulations of ageing, such as brittleness, color changes, and so forth).

In many ways, the pulp in the interior is like the nerve centre of the tooth. It consists of all the structures you would find within living tissue, such as nerves, blood vessels, and connective tissue. The only tissue it lacks is muscle! One of the principal features of pulp is its sensitivity to pain, which is why so many protective layers surround it. In the body, generally, if tissue is hurt, such as if you receive a kick on the shins, it bruises, swells, and inflammation occurs. The body is reacting; all its defenses and repair mechanisms are rushing to the site. If pulp is damaged, it also becomes inflamed. However, it cannot swell up because it is contained within a rigid structure, and the nerves are crushed and become sensitive, resulting in pain. Pain, caused by the transmission of pressure on nerve endings, occurs quickly when the pulp is damaged, and because the outlet, the apical foramen, may be small, this pressure can only be relieved slowly. This explains, to a certain extent, why pain in a tooth can be so severe and seem to persist for such an interminable period.

But teeth are well designed in general, and to protect the pulp from damage, there are further layers: the dentin and the enamel. The layer immediately around the pulp is dentin, which is basically composed of a substance similar to the outer layer, the enamel. Dentin, however, is less hard, of a much more organic composition, a more spaced-out structure in general. It has little tubules that contain mechanisms to register sensations such as pain, whereas the harder enamel is generally thought to be inert. Dentin is similar to bone in composition, but it is structurally different.

Dentin has a further security device, a property completely unique to it—another pointer to the sheer efficiency and farsightedness of the body and its mechanisms. Stone Age man's teeth often wore down quickly because of the abrasive foods he ate. If the enamel wore through, first the dentin and then the pulp would be exposed. To help combat this, and it is still a sign of wear and tear and of ageing in present-day teeth, the tooth lays down more dentin, called "physiological or "adventitious" secondary dentin. This process occurs throughout the life of the tooth and will react to stressful stimuli, such as tooth decay, excessive wear, and pulpal nerve irritation (heat, cold, and chemical). This ensures that there is a longer time span before the attrition causes a painful pulp exposure. Hand in hand with age and this enlarging of the dentin layer goes the diminishing of the size of the pulp chamber.

The outer layer of the tooth, which is the most visible, and therefore the one most people worry about, is the enamel. Enamel is the hardest substance in the body, and its major constituents are calcium and phosphate. It's similar to the material that makes bone, but the calcium for teeth is in a crystalline form, which gives it its hardness. As mentioned before, enamel and dentin are similar in content, although formulated differently: there is 35 percent calcium in enamel, as opposed to 24 percent in dentin; the organic content of enamel is 1.1 percent, as opposed to 21 percent in dentin; there is 4 percent water content in enamel, compared to 10 percent in dentin.[28]

Enamel, although inert, lacks the sensation of pulp and dentin and is not as chemically stable as most people would believe. On the contrary, the surface of the enamel has a certain amount of permeability, meaning that there can be uptake into and loss from that surface, of both good things and bad. The older the tooth, the less permeable it becomes, whereas newly erupted or young teeth are more chemically active, permeable, and therefore vulnerable. Should they be in an environment that produces a lot of acid—a mouth which, sadly, is all too common in the six- to seven-year-old age group, when eating sweets is often at its height—then the acids can attack the permeable enamel much more rapidly and start the process of tooth decay.

However, fluoride is also clinically significant here. Just as the enamel can take up the acids, so can it take up "topical" fluoride—

---

28   Ferguson, D. *Oral Bioscience*. Oxford: Elsevier, Churchill Livingstone 1999, 26.

that is, any fluoride that may be present in the mouth, close to the tooth's surface. As topical fluoride is undoubtedly of benefit to teeth (other less beneficial aspects are discussed elsewhere in this book), the permeability of the enamel can be used to advantage and can help prevent tooth decay. If, for example, a new permanent molar is coated with fluoride shortly after eruption at the age of six or seven, the uptake on the surface will probably be higher; therefore, it will be more effective than it would be on that same tooth if it were left a few years to mature in the mouth.

The final layer in the tooth structure is the cement, which covers the root. The enamel layer normally joins the cement at what is called the "cemento-enamel junction," and this is where the protective cement takes over. If this weren't there, the dentin would be exposed. However, in some 40 percent of the population, the join of the cement does not coincide with the end of the enamel, and there is a little area where the three surfaces—enamel, dentin, and cement—are side by side rather than overlapping. If gums are healthy and firm against the enamel on the side of the tooth, this may not cause too much trouble. If the "seal" between the gum and tooth has been broken—because of incipient gum disease, for example—then the dentin can be stimulated by acidic, sweet, hot or cold foods, or by the toothbrush filaments, and the outcome is commonly known as sensitive teeth. This can also happen with age, as the gums recede, and overly vigorous brushing can also wear away the cement and dentin, as they are not as hard as the enamel.

Calcification

Given the complexity of the structural anatomy of teeth, it is perhaps surprising that there are so few severe problems. But problems undoubtedly do occur, and the major ones involving the actual formation of teeth are those occurring during calcification or mineralization, during the hardening of the teeth. As this hardness is one of the properties unique to them, one of their most useful qualities, any weakening or abnormalities can be disastrous. Hypocalcification (or less calcium than desirable) can result in teeth with irregularities, which can harbor bacteria, with surfaces that are less resistant to tooth decay, and mechanically, they can break and chip more readily.

Teeth are essentially composed of calcium phosphate, and the amount contained in enamel is greater than that found in the underlying dentin or, indeed, in bone. Comparatively speaking, enamel is harder than steel, being virtually the hardest naturally formed substance. The actual composition of tooth is hydroxyapatite, and this has the chemical formula of Ca10 (PO4)6OH. This sounds complicated, but its relevance is such that, as with almost all chemical structures, the formula can be modified by the addition of other elements. There are other inorganic parts of the enamel and dentin, and these, in element form, contain fluoride, lead, zinc, iron, chloride, sodium, magnesium, carbonate, strontium, copper, aluminium, and potassium, to name but a few. Some, such as strontium, fluoride, and zinc, can be relatively high in the tooth composition, while others are more in trace form. Lead, for instance, can show up in the teeth, and one way of testing for a dangerously high intake of lead, or for lead poisoning, might be to examine the shed deciduous teeth of children at risk.

From as early as the third month of pregnancy until the age of eight years, both deciduous and permanent teeth, with the exception of wisdom teeth, are calcifying. During this period, there are factors that may disturb the calcification, and listed below are some examples. Diet is the classic one, and because I consider that so important and so central to my whole thesis, I discuss this separately later on in this chapter.

1. Birth trauma can affect calcification. Birth is an extraordinarily busy time dentally, and there are some forty-four teeth present in the newborn, all in some stage of development, either the crowns or the roots. If the birth process is prolonged, or presents some difficulty or stress to the baby, the calcification is disturbed. Indeed, if you look closely enough at most people's permanent teeth, you can see what we call the neonatal line, a fine line of marginal discoloration in the enamel, which charts the disturbance in the growing of the tooth when the actual birth took place. This line is horizontal to the axis of the tooth,

and it will affect all those teeth that are calcifying at the time of trauma. To illustrate the timing more clearly: at this stage, at birth, the first permanent molars, which don't erupt until about the age of six, are being calcified, and the line will show clearly on them. The effects can also show, particularly if the birth trauma was severe, on the front incisors, and they do not erupt until the age of seven or eight. All births will be stressful to the newborn—and the longer the period of giving birth, the more distinct the neonatal line, i.e., the longer period of time that the process of calcification is disturbed.

1. Antibiotics can affect calcification. The various forms of tetracycline, which are used for sore throats, chest infections, and severe colds, can cause discoloration of the teeth. They are useful antibiotics because, apart from a dental point of view, they don't have many other side effects, but they should not be prescribed for women during pregnancy or lactation, or for a child under the age of eight, by which time calcification is completely finished. These days, in most parts of the world, doctors use alternative antibiotics, as the "tetracycline stain" is a widely known side effect.

   Different forms of tetracycline will produce different colors: aureomycin will produce a gray-brown (either or both); ledermycin, terramycin, and actomycin will produce yellow stains. (Vibromycin is the only one that does not have this discoloring effect.) On the eruption of the tooth and its exposure to ultraviolet light, sunlight, the color change appears. The teeth can also be affected by varying degrees of hypocalcification, so, with less calcium in the tooth than needed, the tooth will be structurally weaker.

2. Calcium is laid down in the teeth in waves, like rings on a tree, with one layer landing on top of another. If a tetracycline is given during this formative time, it tends to target the calcium and thus give a horrendous banding of color right through the layers. This can be disfiguring, and sadly, because it's

incorporated into the teeth rather than lying on the surface, it cannot be polished off. In severe cases, when children are older, the dentist may need to crown the teeth or utilize the veneer techniques that will be discussed later.

3. Another color-change element affecting calcification is fluoride. Those who lobby for the fluoridation of water supplies don't often admit its harmful effect on tooth formation. Fluorine is an element known to deprive the body of calcium, and if ingested excessively during the tooth calcification process, it can interfere with it to a greater or lesser extent.[29]

Fluorosis (the abnormalities caused to the teeth by too much fluoride ingested during this period) is becoming increasingly common in our society. As anything above two parts per million, fluoride to water, is considered potentially hazardous, and with fluoride in drinking water, in toothpastes, in drops, tablets, and topical treatments (it's even contained in tea), many children at the vulnerable stage can be getting far too much.

In mild overdosage, there is a lustreless opaque appearance to the enamel, which should gleam and shine, and it lies either in patches or over the whole tooth. In more severe cases, the teeth can be stained yellow and brown, with mottled enamel creating pits in the surface, which can be havens for bacteria that cause tooth decay. In extreme cases of fluorosis, you can actually get a complete shape change of the tooth as well, with extensive hypoplasia (under calcification). So, although in theory the fluoride may render the tooth more resistant to tooth decay, in reality fluoride can be one of the most serious disfiguring elements for teeth.

If the mother contracts syphilis, she can pass it on to her baby in the womb, and the permanent teeth are more often affected, with deficient or missing enamel, poorly formed dentin, and incisors often shaped rather like crescents. These

[29] Ferguson, D. *Oral Bioscience*. Oxford: Elsevier, Churchill Livingstone 1999, 195–209.

effects of the offspring's teeth will depend on the activity of the disease in the mother during pregnancy. Syphilis is a disease with stages of activity (primary, secondary, and tertiary), with dormant and active spells during the lifespan of the host. However, due to the use of antibiotics and a greater awareness of the dangers of the disease, dentists do not often see patients displaying these signs nowadays.[30]

4. There is a genetic association with abnormal calcification, and this is literally when a family's genes produce bad formation of the tooth structure. Just as a mother's gaps in her teeth might reproduce genetically in her children, so can a parent's tendency to weak teeth or thin enamel be reproduced as well. In amelogenesis imperfecta, the enamel is affected; in dentinogenesis imperfecta, the dentin is affected. This latter condition can almost be worse than damaged enamel: as the underlying structure of the tooth is weak, the tooth can collapse in upon itself once it is used. These are rare conditions.[31]

5. Childhood illnesses such as measles, chicken pox, and scarlet fever, all of which are likely to produce fevers or general disruption in the whole body, will also cause abnormalities if they occur during the years of calcification. Sadly, of course, these years, from birth to about four or five, are the ones in which children most commonly fall prey to a host of ailments. With so many suffering to a greater or lesser degree from colds, snuffles, flu, raised temperatures, and so on, it is therefore not surprising, when looking carefully at the teeth of both older children and adults, that there are so many visible flaws in the enamel, which can then give rise to color inconsistencies. If the illness is long and severe, it can mean the teeth that are calcifying at that time can be virtually ruined.

---

[30] Little, J. "Medline Syphilis: An Update" (Review) (41 Refs). And Putkonen, T. "Medline Dental Changes in Congenital Sypilis; Relationship to Other Syphilitic Stigmata" *Acta Dermato-Venereologica*, 42: 44–62, 1962.

[31] Crawford, P. Ameogensis Imperfecta (AI) and Dentinogensis Imperfecta (DI), www.dentalschool.bris.ac.uk.

6. The final thing that can commonly affect calcification is local infection or trauma. This occurs at a later stage, in the first two years, for example, and a classic instance is when a child falls over and damages his front baby teeth, pushing them up in the jaw. If they ascend far enough, this can physically affect the germ of the permanent tooth above, and if this is not fully calcified at the time, it will be damaged. Similarly, if a child gets early tooth decay, such as with a dental abscess on a baby tooth, the development of the permanent tooth above or beneath can be affected as well.

Nutrition and Calcification

To put it simply, correct nutrition is the foundation of health for the whole body, including the teeth. A good maternal diet during pregnancy and lactation, and for the child, especially during that estimated four-year calcification period, is an investment for the whole future of the child and of his teeth. At no other time does growth take place quite so quickly as in the womb and in the first years of life, and so it is of paramount importance that the body cells obtain the maximum support and help from food, which is, of course, what is required to make them grow.

A good diet will ensure that jaws and other bones of the body can achieve their maximum potential, that teeth are well formed, and that calcification is as complete as possible. An additional benefit can be good general health, which will lessen the vulnerability to infections of all kinds for both mother and child. This should remove many of the causes of calcification abnormalities mentioned above. General health and good formation of teeth will also lessen the susceptibility to tooth decay, because well-formed teeth and jaws are more resistant to disease.

Calcium phosphate is the major constituent of both tooth and bone; about 99 percent of the calcium in our bodies is in bones and teeth (the rest is for proper contraction of the muscles), and fortunately calcium is commonly found in food (even processed convenience foods). Unless a diet is very peculiar or unbalanced, it's not often

Great Teeth for Life

that there is a serious deprivation, but we can occasionally find effects on teeth that are the direct result of insufficient calcium in the diet. Those most at risk are growing children and pregnant or lactating mothers. If the mother's diet is low in calcium, she may lose calcium from her bones, not from her teeth. There may be a greater likelihood of gum disease, but this is brought about by hormonal changes rather than by calcium loss, as is commonly believed. The baby will not suffer as soon as the mother—its demands have priority—but in extreme deprivation of calcium, poor skull and bone development, as well as poor teeth, can be a result.[32]

Calcium is contained in such diverse things as milk and other dairy products (cheese and yogurt particularly) and canned sardines. Milk, of course, is what is normally recommended for pregnant mothers so that they may build up their calcium reserves. I believe, though, along with other nutritional practitioners, that the calcium in cows' milk is often not in the best form for easy digestion, and the milk itself contains additives, so it may not be the best source. Green leafy vegetables and other vegetables such as carrots, as well as whole grains, also contain calcium, and they should provide adequate supplies.

The average daily uptake of calcium is 0.02oz (0.8 grams), while pregnant and lactating women require about 0.5-0.7oz (1.5–2 grams). The overall amount of calcium in a newborn baby is 25 grams. From birth to about ten months, it goes up to 43 grams; by the end of the first year, there's a massive leap to 83 grams, illustrating dramatically that during periods of rapid growth (pregnancy and that first year), there is a much larger requirement for calcium.[33] Fortunately, those extra needs are met by the body, which can extract greater amounts of the mineral from food eaten.

32 Fish, E. *An Experimental Investigation on Enamel, Dentin and the Dental Pulp.* London: John Bale Sons & Danielsson, Ltd., 1933. Rasmussen, P. "Calcium Deficiency, Pregnancy and Lactation, Norway," *J Periodontal Res.*, 12(4); 283–289.

33 Atkinson, P.J., West R.R., "Loss of Skeletal Calcium in Lactating Women," J. *Obstet Gynaecol Br Commonw* 1970
Chistiansen C., Rodbro P., Heinild B., *Unchanged Total Body Calcium in Normal Human Pregnancy*, Acta Obstet Gynecol Scand., 1976.
Duggin, G.G. et al, Calcium Balance in Pregnancy, Lancet 1974,19, p. 926-927.

Thus, the amount of absorption from the stomach and the amount that is actually utilized by the body can be regulated in such times of need. In fact, all animals, including children, absorb greater proportions of calcium when growing, and even adults apparently vary their calcium uptake seasonally—an interesting thought that might be a throwback to when diet might change seasonally, when there might not be enough food through the winter, or perhaps something to do with breeding cycles. Indeed, during the latter months of human pregnancy, of the extra amount of calcium that is absorbed, only half goes into the baby: the other half goes into the bones of the mother.[34] We presume that this is in order to provide a reserve for lactation because bones can effectively store calcium and other minerals. Hormonal changes actually will alter the uptake of calcium, so again it is a controlled mechanism.

The main problem with calcium is absorption, and only part of what we eat is absorbed. It all depends yet again on good diet in general and certain vitamins in particular. An unbalanced diet can lead to malabsorption, so even though a mother, for example, might be having the right quantity of calcium in her diet, because of other dietary factors leading to a wrong combination in her body, that calcium will be inadequately absorbed.

Vitamin D is essential for the mechanism controlling absorption of calcium (as well as for the metabolism). It occurs in relatively few foods. Fish, margarine, eggs, dairy foods, liver, and cod liver oil—which used to be the bane of many a child's life—are the major sources. Fortunately, our skin manufactures vitamin D when exposed to sunlight, and though the summer months typically supply us with a certain proportion of our vitamin D requirements, we often need to rely upon our diets the rest of the year. Asians and West Indians living in Britain, whose dark skins were designed to protect them from stronger sunlight, are not able to manufacture vitamin D in the weaker northern sunlight, so they may need vitamin D supplements. Older people also sometimes suffer from lack of vitamin D: they wrap themselves up, stay inside to keep warm, and don't get enough sunshine as a result.

---

34 Paterson, C. "Calcium Requirements in Man: A Critical Review." *Postgrad Med.* 1978 April, 244–248.

A deficiency of vitamin D in general, because it is so vital in the absorption and use of calcium, can cause bones to become brittle and teeth to be ultimately lost. Vitamin D is the substance most closely associated with rickets and osteomalacia, which means that when a child stands, the leg bones can bend and cause permanent deformity. Dentally, with a serious vitamin D deficiency, teeth can be badly formed (hypoplastic). Research has also suggested[35] that vitamin D can help prevent tooth decay. It may be that vitamin D, present in the saliva, enhances the oral environment and lessens the chances of decay developing.

Vitamins A and C, as well as other minerals such as magnesium, zinc, and many trace elements, are also vital to the calcification process, as they are to health generally. But it must be emphasized, though, that it is all a matter of balance, with a correct combination, and the only way this can be truly ensured is through a correct and sensible diet.

A number of things can interfere in a dietary sense with the absorption of calcium, and thus with the calcification process. Rickets and osteomalacia, direct results of defects with calcium metabolism in the tissues, can be found in Britain in some children from the Indian subcontinent[36]. It is thought that this may be because the diet in these areas includes a large proportion of chapatti, a basic bread made from hard whole-wheat flour. This flour is high in phytates, which slow the absorption of calcium and can actually "suck" calcium from the body, along with other minerals like magnesium. Research has shown that when chapatti was removed from their diet for a period as short as seven weeks, there was a marked rise in the calcium levels in their bodies.[37] This is interesting in showing how a diet based on one food in large proportions can have a deleterious effect on the body, but even more so when one considers recent fads like high-roughage diets. Dietary fiber is undeniably essential for health, but an overemphasis on the basics of such a diet, including

---

35   Nick, G., Hoffman, R. "Vitamin D Deficiency and Tooth Decay, Whole Health Source: Reversing Tooth Decay," Whole Health Source, blogspot.com/2009
36   Osteomalacia (Soft Bones) www.arc.org.uk/arthinfo/patpubs
37   Clements M. "The Problem of Rickets in UK Asians." J Hum Nutri, 1989, 105–16.

brown rice, brown bread, and especially bran—all of which are high in phytates—can have a marked effect on the body. Although the body, being an adaptable organ, can become accustomed to a high phytate diet, there is quite a large and rapid drain of calcium at first. The main significance is that dangers could lie in overenthusiastic parents putting their growing children on such a diet. Calcium loss at such a time would be hazardous, and immature digestive systems would not be able to cope anyway.

Another factor affecting calcium absorption is the oxalic acid contained in foods such as spinach and rhubarb. Despite Popeye, and the powers given him by spinach, both foods should be avoided or at least limited in the diets of growing children and expectant mothers.[38] While raw, fresh organically grown spinach is a superb whole food, cooking it creates the active acid that prevents the absorption of essential minerals.

Finally, with regard to diet and calcification, studies show[39] that a high-protein diet can help the absorption of calcium, as can the sugar or lactose in breast milk. I'm not necessarily recommending high-protein consumption, but it has some value in this area, although it also aids the excretion of calcium. But I am unreservedly recommending breastfeeding, as mother's milk is by far the best food any baby can have, not least because it will help in the calcification process and is a whole food.

The Jaw

From the dental point of view, the jaw is the foundation stone, so to speak, of the whole dental configuration, and without its efficient working movements—opening, closing, and chewing—many would not be able to survive. If food is not chewed properly, it affects the whole digestive system. It has been shown that when

---

38 Zarembski, P.; Hodgkinson, A. "The Oxalic Acid Content of English Diets," Brit J Nutri 1962, 16, 627, www.revolutionhealth.com/drugs-treatments/low-oxalate-diet

39 The Effect of Protein on Calcium Absorption and Gastric Acid Production, Dec 22, 2008, Clinical Trials, Gov. Information provided by Yale University, Connecticut, USA.

food is placed directly into the stomach, the experimental animal will become ill. If the same food is then chewed thoroughly in the mouth, taken out and placed in the stomach, the animal recovers its health.

Interestingly, just as teeth have priority over bone and even in severe nutritional crises do not easily yield their minerals (thus, accordingly, their hardness), nature has also built safeguards into the jaw. Although we tend to think of babies as being quite helpless, unlike most other animal babies, they do still have certain birth reflexes. The Moro reflex is one. This occurs when a baby, thinking he is about to be dropped, jerkily splays his limbs and grabs with his hands—an echo, it is thought, of when the baby clung to his mother's fur. The fisting of the baby's hands around a finger is another reflex. Dentally, though, the jaw will automatically open and close without any control from the upper brain. A baby does not have to be taught to suck or chew, for the instinct is already there. In fact, even if all the nerves that control the jaw were cut in an accident, for example, with the victim a virtual living vegetable, the body would still react instinctively to the stimulation of something between the lips and teeth, and would open, close, and chew (albeit only after a fashion). Nourishment of the body has priority yet again.

The jaw begins to form in the fetus even earlier than the teeth, from about the fourth week after conception. Certainly before any knowledge of pregnancy, the tissue which will become the arches of the jaw and palates is growing. Specialized cells known as osteoblasts and osteoclasts model the growth and formation of the jaw after a baby is born, and throughout the child's entire growing period. The former make the bone grow and deposit bone, and the latter dissolve bone. These cells are stimulated to make the teeth move through the jaw, both in the transition from deciduous to permanent teeth, and in the period when orthodontic treatments, braces, and other dental appliances may have to play a part. This constant activity and mobility means that the alveolar bones in the jaw, the ones that actually hold the teeth in place, are much more flexible than an adult's and remain so throughout the entire growing period. This flexibility comes in handy when children go through their falling over and bumping faces period. They don't do nearly as much damage as an adult undergoing the same trauma might, and this may be nature's way of compensating for those years of instability and accidents.

Shaping of the Jaws

What forms the nice arcs of the upper and lower jaws and teeth?

This is due to the lips and tongue, which act like physical barriers to contain the teeth: the tongue pushes the teeth outwards towards the lip, and the lips and cheeks push the teeth inwards towards the tongue. For example, if a growing child had only part of a tongue, then the teeth and jawbone on that side would tend to veer towards the area that had no tissue to push them out again (a malformation of this basic shaping mechanism can occur with a thumb sucker, who will pull the top teeth out and push the bottom ones in). Even a baby who lies on one side all the time can depress that side of the face and jaw so that it may look a little lopsided for a while, but this will normally correct itself. Another basic shaping factor is breastfeeding. Proper sucking from the breast, the system designed by nature, will promote the best shape and development of the jaw and facial bone structure, and of the facial musculature in general. Where breastfeeding is not possible, modern dummies and teats have been designed to assist the correct growth of the jaws during this vital formative period.

Some major factors controlling jaw and teeth are still thought to be genetic, inherited from the parents: the size of the jaw, the shape, the size of the teeth, and whether they are well spaced within the jaw. A father's gap between his front teeth can be reproduced in his children, as can a mother's square or pointed chin and jaw. The class of jaw can be inherited too. This is of significance dentally in orthodontics, and refers to the bite of the teeth, how the upper and lower teeth come together in the jaw. Class 1 is where the teeth meet virtually edge to edge. Class 2 is where the top teeth protrude beyond the bottom teeth, and class 3 is where the bottom teeth stick out beyond the top teeth. Class 1, is generally considered to be the ideal, but in fact it is rare in Western civilization to have a

Great Teeth for Life

normal occlusion, to use the dental term. Jaw class can also run in families. One of the most famous is that of the Habsburgs, the most prominent European imperial dynasty from the fifteenth to the twentieth centuries. From portraits, we can clearly see the classic class 3, or lantern, jaw. But class of jaw can also be a racial characteristic. Many Chinese or Japanese people have class 2 bites and a slight class 3 is quite commonly seen in Scottish people!

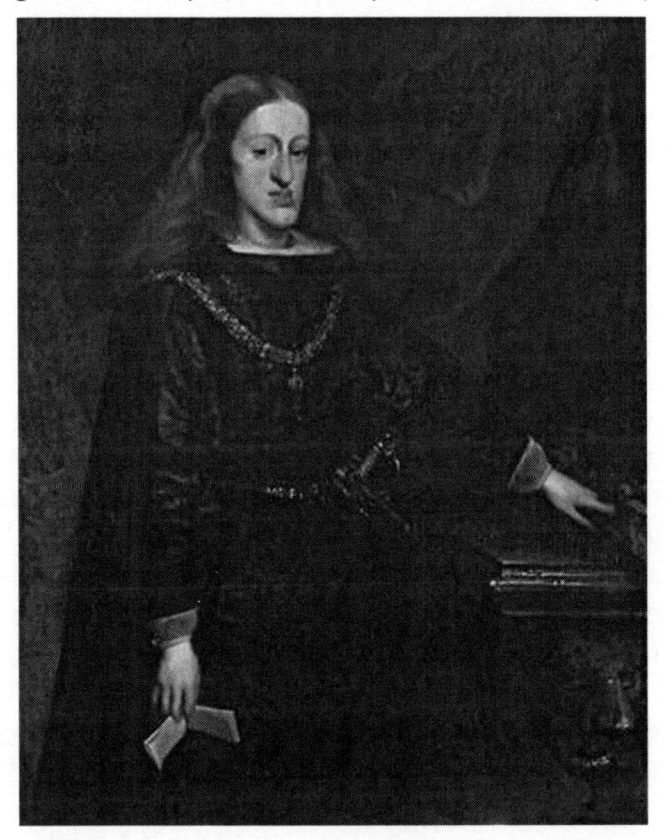

Fig. 11
The Habsburg Jaw—Portrait of Charles II of Spain and Provence
This is a faithful photographic reproduction of an original two-dimensional work of art. The work of art itself is in the public domain because its copyright has expired. This applies to the United States, Australia, the European Union, and those countries with a copyright term of life of the author plus seventy years.

When genetic or racial types are mixed, problems can occur dentally. A father with a large jaw and teeth together with a mother with a small jaw and small teeth can produce a child with a small jaw and large teeth. If large teeth are crammed together in a jaw too small to accommodate them properly, the child will be prey to all the problems that are associated with crowded teeth, including difficulty in cleaning properly between tight teeth, and thus a vulnerability to bacterial invasion, followed by tooth decay and gum disease.

This genetic aspect of jaw shape and its relationship with tooth crowding was taught to me as an undergraduate at dental school and was considered to be virtually the only cause of tooth crowding and therefore a major contributory factor to tooth decay. Although much was taught on the relationship between tooth decay and diet, there was little consideration of the relationship between diet and crowded jaws. That no further significant research has been done on this subject, some seventy years after the findings of Dr. Weston Price, an American dentist, seems unbelievable to me. As mentioned previously, his book *Nutrition and Physical Degeneration* was published in the 1930s, and it has become a bible, the foundation stone, for many nutritionists the world over. Dr. Price investigated fourteen primitive peoples worldwide, peoples who were purebred, who had little contact with the outside world, and who were living on traditional tribal unprocessed and unrefined foods. They included Australian Aborigines, Alaskans, Polynesians, Eskimos, and people living in remote Swiss valleys and in the high mountains of Peru, and although there was an enormous diversity of races, tribal customs, and native foods, Dr. Price observed perfect teeth and good jaw and skeletal structures everywhere.

He found a great change in these people, however, after they came in contact with civilization and with "civilized" foods—white sugar and flour, etc.—after one generation only, and the effects exhibited themselves with horrifying rapidity. The people were suffering quite visibly from tooth decay and from a narrowing of jaws and dental arches. His book is filled with before and after photographs, which illustrate dramatically, with no possible doubt, how damaging modern refined foods can be, and how inextricably linked nutrition and dental health are.

Great Teeth for Life

The first important fact about Dr. Price's work is its unique timeliness. Historically speaking, the decade in which he made and reported his findings was undoubtedly the last in which anyone had an opportunity to study such isolated communities. For one can no longer find any part of the world in which the peoples and their diets have not been basically altered, to a greater or lesser extent, by the "advances" of civilization: refined foods, fertilizers, drugs and chemicals, or by pollution. Even in the 1930s, he encountered these people on the cusp, so to speak, being able to record their health verbally and photographically, both dentally and generally, before and after the introduction of modern ideas and foods.

The second factor that I consider vital is that he recorded so many different races. He did not look at just one or two peoples who perhaps were physiologically weaker or stronger, or who geographically were able to enjoy a better or worse diet (Eskimos ate meat almost exclusively; some had a mixed diet; some were virtually vegetarian). He looked at a huge variety in every sense, and everywhere he noted superlative health, which then degenerated in an astonishingly short time. He was looking at generation upon generation of purebred people, people who were not affected by the crossbreeding of racial types found in the Northern Hemisphere generally. In all cases, he recorded good dental arches, good facial formations, broad nasal arches, and wide jaws, yet within ten to fifteen years, these had all changed, and many of the younger people looked as if they belonged to a different tribe.[40]

With the introduction of modern food, the sugars particularly, the first deterioration was that of tooth decay. The second most noticeable factor was that the developing children then suffered from malocclusions or bad growth of the jaws, with teeth crowded as a result. This occurred almost immediately, not just in the womb, but exhibiting itself also in three- and four-year-olds, who, by the time they were twelve, were showing crowding, decay, and jaw degeneration that had never before been seen in their family or group. Many also exhibited a rapid deterioration in their resistance to disease. In this pre-antibiotic era, tuberculosis was endemic, but

---

40   Genepool –wikipedia "genetic diversity" National/biological/ information infrastructure. NBII 16 March 2008 www.nbii.gov

because of a good natural resistance, it was not common in these isolated communities. Dr. Price recorded that those children who showed severe jaw degeneration also had antisocial and behavioral changes.

Some of his conclusions can, with justification, be criticized, due to the decade in which he was working. His grasp of the interaction of vitamins and minerals was good, but in the late 1930s, he lacked knowledge of the detailed research that has gone on since. In general, however, he shows in an extraordinarily graphic way the profound effect that diet can have on health, raising horrifying questions: If undeniably strong genetic bases can be so visibly affected, and so rapidly, by diet, what about the changes that cannot be so easily registered? What might be happening to the body internally?

CHAPTER FOUR

You Are What You Eat—and What Your Parents Ate Too!

How can we guarantee that our children have good teeth? And where do we start? If dentistry becomes primarily preventative, as I hope most sincerely it does, then good advice must be given from the very beginning, and the parents must take the utmost care of their children, from that initial twinkle in the father's eye onward. It is the only way in which we can ensure the health of future generations.

Preconceptual Care

It seems to me one of life's greatest ironies that although commercial livestock and show animal breeders, even hamster breeders, believe in a special program and diets before breeding to ensure normal and healthy young, future human parents do not seem to give much thought to the health of their own bodies in relation to that of their potential offspring. Only in primitive societies, many of which were studied by Dr. Weston Price, do we find any real evidence of this preconceptual concern. He recorded that in many different races, when a couple reached an age where they were thinking of having children, they were often put on special diets and given the best meats and the best and freshest foods in general. Thus, they could be both more fertile, and their sperm and ovum would have the best nutrition possible in order, hopefully, to produce the strongest offspring. They believed—and in the light of present-day knowledge, how can we deny it?—that they could help improve the quality of the species and produce a better and healthier next generation.

It goes without saying that the healthier the parents have been throughout their lives, and the healthier they are in the months prior to conception, then the healthier the baby. Many nutritionists nowadays believe that the bodies of both father and mother should be primed for at least two years prior to conception, and at the forefront of research and practice in Britain is Foresight, the Association for the Promotion of Preconceptual Care (www.foresight-preconception.org.uk). The thinking behind Foresight has largely been inspired by the research of Dr. Weston Price in the 1930s, but the conclusions have been put strongly and ably into practice on a much more scientific basis. Instead of totally relying upon the principles of good diet, although these are central to their aims and to the advice given by them, they also undertake many tests on prospective parents who attend their clinics.

A full medical history is taken and relevant factors are noted, like allergies, illnesses, forms of contraception used, and whether the mother has had German measles. They take all the usual tests and perform a hair analysis. (The latter, important for fathers as well, can give a good insight into mineral and metal levels and deficiencies during the three or so months of the hair growth.) They even monitor other environmental factors such as drinking water, checking water at both home and work if hair samples have shown any metal contamination in excess of the World Health Organization limits. Foresight also recommends preconceptual supplements for both parents, marketing three different varieties, which contain a wide range of vitamins and minerals, and publishes helpful leaflets. By this general health screening, of course, defects that could hamper fertility or cause defects in a future baby can be brought to light, examined, referred on to general medical practitioners or specialists, and remedied if possible before conception.

A planned pregnancy is the most sensible of all, for before a mother even realizes she has missed her first period, she may have encountered many substances, whether environmental or dietary, that might be harmful to the growing child. For it must never be forgotten that during the first six to eight weeks after conception, all the organs of the body, limbs, face, jaw, and teeth begin their separate development. I feel that this preconceptual care is vital, and holistic dentists could play a significant part in this area. If newly married couples came, for example, to the dentist to be checked, the dentist could ask them if they were thinking of starting a family. If the answer was affirmative, he could offer them advice and give them some health pointers. He could provide literature on nutrition or refer them to an organization like Foresight. He might even ultimately be enabled to do some of the tests himself. The dentist, seeing people at regular intervals, is in an extremely strong position to monitor general health, and to step in with significant advice at such appropriate times.

Pointers to Preconceptual Health

1. If a prospective mother has not had German measles, she should be immunized against the disease at least three months before conception. This avoids the risks of babies being born with hearing and other defects.

2. If a prospective mother is taking an oral contraceptive pill, she should change to an alternative method of contraception at least four to six months before planning to conceive in order to reduce risk of miscarriage and defects (the pill also reduces the mother's levels of vitamin C and iron). Those using the copper coil should change contraceptive method at about the same time.

3. If drugs are taken in connection with diseases such as diabetes, eczema, asthma, migraine, or epilepsy, then the parents, especially the mother, should seek a doctor's advice at least three months before conception. As drug taking should be completely avoided during pregnancy, advance consideration should be given to the alternatives. Foresight also advises in this area.

4. If the parents smoke, particularly the mother, they should try to stop before conception. The physical manifestations of

nicotine withdrawal, as well as the psychological ones, can be distressing, so it is more sensible to do this immediately. It should most particularly be avoided during pregnancy, but as it so profoundly affects all the cells and tissue of the body, it can only do good to cut it out at this stage.

5. Follow a sensible organic whole food diet (see "Dietary Guidelines," page 187), avoiding as much as possible any excesses, such as alcohol. At least five portions of fresh fruit and vegetables, preferably raw, should be eaten daily; they are rich in vitamins and minerals. Less fatty protein sources such as liver, poultry, and fish should be eaten two or three times a week. Eat plenty of whole grains, nuts, and pulses (lentils, peas, beans, etc.). For snacks, eat dried fruits as opposed to sweets or cakes. If unable to obtain organic, then you should choose locally produced, fresh, and *whole* foods. Avoid genetically produced food and any food with many additives— i.e., read the label! Remember, quality not quantity. Avoid obesity. Remember also to try to boost the calcium reserves even at this stage. Avoid fat as much as possible, whether the type that is visible on meat, or that which is hidden in butter, some cheeses, whole milks, etc. Avoid salt as much as possible—and sugar at all costs!

6. Mothers should get as much exercise as they can in the months prior to pregnancy. Exercise of any kind tones up the body in general and benefits the heart and lungs in particular. Gentle floor or yoga exercises are particularly helpful for relaxing mind and body. Remember that anything now is valuable, but seek advice from your doctor, pediatric practitioner, or trainer as to the amount and type of exercise, as too much exercise during the actual pregnancy can sometimes be harmful. Fresh air is important too, for oxygen is as much a nutrient of the body as good food is.

Prenatal Care

Once conception has taken place, the onus is on the mother to make her body the most ideal environment in which the baby can grow and flourish to its fullest potential. More than at any other time, her diet is absolutely crucial, for what she ingests will pass through her body to the baby. Teeth and bone structure, general mental and physical health, freedom from allergies, and intellectual potential, although to an extent governed by heredity, are mainly dependent upon maternal diet during the nine months spent in the womb.[41] The womb environment can also be damaged or modified, however, by factors other than diet, and the mother has to constantly maintain her scrupulous guardianship of her growing baby.

Once again, the dentist could be at the forefront of medical care at this stage. A dentist's knowledge of a patient's pregnancy is vital anyway, in a number of ways. As dental work is free in Britain during pregnancy and for a year afterward, many mothers take advantage of that fact and attend more regularly. Because pregnancy does undoubtedly cause some mothers distinct dental problems, they will probably need to consult the dentist. However, X-rays are thought to be hazardous to the growing baby, so the dentist will have to be informed before undertaking any treatment involving X-rays.

On no account should existing amalgam fillings be disturbed or placed in a pregnant or lactating woman.[42] Amalgam fillings are mainly composed of silver and mercury. Disturbing old amalgam (mercury fillings) will release mercury vapor. Certain kinds of fish should also be avoided (e.g., tuna, shark, swordfish) because they contain high levels of mercury. A dentist could also give dietary

---

41 (a) Guvyaa Wu et al., "Maternal Nutrition and Foetal Development." The American Society for Nutritional Sciences, Sept 2004.
(b) www.tjclarkinc.com—Pregnancy and Nutrition
(c) Langley-Evans, S., ed. *Fetal Nutrition and Adult Disease: Programming of Chronic Disease through Foetal Exposure to Undernutrition (Frontiers in Nutritional Science* series), Oxfordshire: CABI, 2004
42 The American College of Obstetricians and Gynecologists (ACOG)

advice and keep an eye on how the patient and patient-to-be is progressing. Health care in general at this time is very good, with doctors, antenatal clinics, and health visitors monitoring and contributing health and dietary advice.

Although an organization like Foresight is available, a nutritionally trained dentist could play a part. Indeed, there is no reason why the same advice should not come from all sources—the more the merrier, in fact. It's indubitably true of life, but particularly true when you're a first-time mother, that the greater the number of professional people who agree on a subject relating to you—in this case, a good diet—the more likely you are to follow that advice, and the more assured you will be that you are doing the right thing.

The dentist could be utilized much more as yet another health screen, so to speak. If he has a good relationship with his patient, often a relaxed conversation between them can clear up many a point thought to be too trivial to bother a doctor with. If he keeps a full medical history of his patient, and I believe every dentist should, then he can reassure and back up normal medical advice about such things as high blood pressure, diabetes, and so on. He could be the one to spot anemia or some vitamin deficiency in a pregnant patient, and he might also spot weight abnormalities. He could look out for some of the danger signs such as alcoholism, smoking, or drug taking, and he could give advice on such maternal vagaries as pica, the craving for eating inedible substances such as coal! With so many teenage pregnancies these days, he could advise on diet, for the teenage proclivity for hamburgers and fizzy drinks could be detrimental to the health of mother and baby, as well as the teeth and gums of the expectant mum.

A Healthy Diet During Pregnancy

That good maternal diet is essential to produce a healthy baby, both bodily and dentally, is undisputed at every level of medical practice. In fact, there is a definite relationship between poor nutrition and the poor physical growth of the fetus, especially in the development of the lower brain section, which is associated with coordination

Great Teeth for Life

and general physical ability. The teeth, as already outlined, take priority over bone when there are dietary deficiencies.

The mother's own long-term health is dependent on her diet at this time too, and there is no reason why she should lose her teeth through gum disease, as well as her figure, and end up with unsightly varicose veins, stretch marks, and wrinkles.[43] There is no need either, despite the old belief, to "eat for two," which would lead to an unnecessary weight gain that is difficult to shed afterward. A certain gain is necessary to allow for the growth of the baby, the fat deposits to be used for breastfeeding, for the placenta and amniotic fluid, etc.

The average total gain required is about eighteen pounds (eight kilograms), and more than twenty to twenty-four pounds (nine to twelve kilograms) would indicate undesirable excess fat or fluid retention. The need during pregnancy is for increased nutrients, not increased calories; even in midterm, a mother only needs about an extra three hundred calories a day, and extra bulk, like sweet buns, can only have a detrimental effect on the mother's teeth and her figure after birth. And it won't do the baby any good.

Although I go on below to specify many vitamins and minerals that are desirable for bodily and dental health at this time, I must emphasize that the overall balance of the diet is what's important. If the mother eats the right foods and carefully considers them in relationship with each other, all the necessities will be ingested in the most natural way, thus obviating the need for supplementation.

Many pregnant mothers used to be given supplements of iron. They undoubtedly need iron during pregnancy, as the baby has to take enough from its mother to see it through the months in the womb and the first few months of life, and too little iron in the diet could thus lead to maternal anemia. However, at the same time, too much iron, when there is tablet supplementation, for example, could interfere with the absorption and use of other minerals and

---

43   ACOG Education Pamphlet APOOI, Nutrition During Pregnancy.

trace elements such as magnesium and zinc, which are equally as important.[44]

Although pregnancy can be a time when constipation is a problem, overenthusiastic consumption of bran or other high-fiber foods can diminish vitamin D and calcium absorption. Balance must be the key word, and if it sounds as if you should have a biochemistry degree before giving birth, don't worry: follow a few simple rules and rely on a good healthy diet, which should do it all for you!

Proteins

These are required for growth and repair of all the organs of the body, and most people in the Northern Hemisphere probably get more than enough. The approximate daily protein requirement[45] of an expectant mother is about two ounces (50 grams), and that is contained in a couple of slices of good wholemeal bread or a cup of milk. An eight-ounce steak (225 grams) is an overindulgence. Too much meat during pregnancy can mean too large of a phosphorus intake, which can lead to leg cramps. A full range of proteins (which are composed of a complete range of amino acids, the constituents of protein), is found in milk (human, animal, and dried), meat, poultry, fish, eggs, cheese, yogurt, and soya beans (the only food of non-animal origin that is a complete protein). Incomplete proteins supplying a limited range of amino acids are contained in whole grains and all products made from them—such as pasta and bread—and in dried beans, peas, lentils, etc., as well as in nuts and seeds.

I believe that many sources of complete protein should be questioned, for it's the quality of the food that counts. Meats nowadays contain additives, and the meat-producing animals are given growth hormones. Milk and cheese also contain additives.

---

44   www.babycentre.co.uk/pregnancy/complications/anaemia   Anaemia (iron deficiency)

45   King, J. "Energy and Protein Requirements During Pregnancy." University of California, Berkeley, USA, for Joint Food and Agriculture of UN, WHO, United Nations University, 1981

Eggs and poultry should be free-range, and fish is perhaps the only source of protein that is still relatively free of tampering, although pollution is already taking its toll. Vegetables, however, if grown organically and unsprayed, will supply good protein, and a variety of the incomplete proteins will see most expectant mothers, especially vegetarians who need to be particularly careful to have sufficient protein, happily through pregnancy. Any of the above proteins, if genuinely organically produced, will give the correct nutritional balance.

Fats

Expectant moms should be careful about fat consumption, but a moderate amount is needed during pregnancy. Research suggests[46] that essential fatty acids needed in tooth formation may be provided by fish oils and unheated olive, sunflower, and safflower oils, etc., but the major role of fats and oils in diet, and particularly at this stage, is that they are responsible for the absorption of the fat-soluble vitamins A, D, E, and K. Again, all sources of fat should be organic.

Vitamins

The necessity for vitamin D has already been discussed. The other vitamins given as drops to babies are vitamins A and C, and they are important dentally during pregnancy. Vitamin A is important for the formation of tooth enamel and for the connective tissue or collagen. A vitamin A deficiency can affect the osteoblasts, the cells that deposit or make bone, thus teeth, jaws, and other bones are affected. In one form, vitamin A is contained in animal and fish livers (cod liver oil is the major source) and dairy foods. In a second form, it is found in beta-carotene, in green, yellow, and orange vegetables

---

46 Encyclopaedia Britannica, www.britannica.com/EBchecked/topic/nutrition/nutrients

and fruit (carrots, spinach, and dried apricots in particular). Vitamin A, like vitamin D, is poisonous in too large doses.

Vitamin C (ascorbic acid) cannot be manufactured in the human body, although of course we can ingest it. Animals can manufacture vitamin C. Dr. Weston Price, when studying peoples who lived in the snowy wastes of the north, found that in the absence of fruit and vegetables, Eskimos learned to eat certain glands (the adrenals) of the animals they killed, which contained vitamin C. Ascorbic acid is involved in tooth formation and is vital in the building of tissue structures such as collagen. It is strongly linked with iron. A lack of vitamin C during pregnancy can intervene with the function of osteoblasts. As mentioned earlier, a severe deficiency of vitamin C is called scurvy. Babies can develop a form of scurvy, which basically exhibits itself as bleeding gums, and there can also be gross swelling and ulceration in the mouth. Regular doses (one thousand milligrams) of vitamin C can prevent mouth ulcers and reduce gum disease in adults.

Vitamin C is found in fresh fruit and vegetables, and it is water-soluble. Heat destroys vitamin C, so it should be avoided whenever possible. Although this vitamin is undeniably important, it should not be taken in supplemental doses during pregnancy (RDA is seventy milligrams) unless under medical supervision.[47] The baby could actually suffer after birth from vitamin C withdrawal, believe it or not. With such a high level of the vitamin circulating while it was in the womb, it could develop a low vitamin C level and scurvy symptoms in the months after birth. I advise women to stick to organic fresh fruit and vegetables for adequate requirements of vitamin C during pregnancy.

The vitamin B group, including B1 (thiamin), B2 (riboflavin), nicotinic acid (niacin in the United States), pantothenic acid, B6 (pyridoxine), B12 (cyanocobalamine), and folic acid, are all important requirements during pregnancy, major sources being yeast extract, wheat germ, and liver. Deficiencies of some of these can affect the mouth and tongue. In pregnancy, however, a deficiency of B6 and B12 can cause anemia, but a proper intake of B6 can reduce nausea,

---

47   www.drugsafetysite.com/vitamin-c/

Great Teeth for Life

fatigue, dizziness, and leg cramps. Vitamin B12 does not occur in plants in large amounts, and thus vegetarian mothers should take supplements.

Folic acid is perhaps the most important vitamin B, though, for a deficiency has been shown to be a major causative factor in spina bifida and other malformations of the fetus. Foods rich in folic acid should be eaten before conception and after, especially in the first weeks of pregnancy, so that there is a sufficient level circulating in those vital first stages of embryo development, the time when there is the greatest risk that abnormalities may occur. Mothers who have been on the pill before pregnancy, and those who have had several children in close proximity, have particularly high needs for high folic acid levels. Some wheat germ on a daily basis is ample, but a good mnemonic is "folic, foliate, foliage," thus dark green vegetables! Cook them lightly for, like vitamin C, folic acid is destroyed by boiling (keep the vegetable water for soups and sauces).

Vitamin E is thought to be helpful[48] during the labor itself, so a diet rich in it, wheat germ, vegetable oils, and peanuts is good as a preparation! Vitamin E supplements should *not* be taken.

Vitamin K is needed for the clotting of blood, essential in childbirth, and a new baby will have low levels. Dark green vegetables like cabbage, sprouts, spring greens, and broccoli are the best sources.

Minerals and Trace Elements

Minerals such as calcium, phosphorus, iron, potassium, zinc, and sodium are essential for the health and growth of the body. Trace elements such as magnesium, selenium, manganese iodine, and chromium, to name a few, are also of great importance for the body to grow and thrive. Most commercially grown food is grown or fed

---

48 http://www.pregnancy-bliss.co.uk/vitaminsinpregnancy.html. Reuters "Too much vitamin E during pregnancy may harm baby"; source BJOG (International Journal of Obstetrics and Gynecology Feb 2009)

from depleted soils,[49] and therefore you should eat organic produce wherever possible. The modern alternative may be to consider well-formulated supplements.

The above are all the basic constituents of a good diet, but balance must be remembered. If a mother chooses fresh vegetables and fruit, keeps her meat intake low, and cuts out all processed or refined foods, sugars, and salt completely, her health and that of her baby can be assured. If genuine organic foods are consumed, many of the worries of "Am I or my baby getting all the essential nutrients for good health?" are answered.

Maternal Teeth during Pregnancy

During pregnancy, there are major upheavals in the body, especially hormone levels. Hormones can affect the gums, giving rise to pregnancy gingivitis. Suffice to say that if nutrition is poor, with a deficiency of calcium or zinc, for example, then any disease process already present in the mouth will be magnified.

One of the other difficulties encountered at this time concerns pregnancy nausea or sickness and tooth decay. The advice given by many authorities is to eat small but frequent meals in order to avert nausea. Dentally, however, this can cause tooth decay, for it is the frequency of sugar, for example, that is much more damaging than the quantity. By having a high-quality diet, most mothers wouldn't be taking much sugar anyway, but a good precaution during the nine months would be to brush teeth correctly after every meal, as this will also help keep gum disease at bay. Visits to the dental hygienist should be more frequent during pregnancy for obvious reasons.

---

49   (a) James W. Lyne et al. "Are Depleted Soils Causing a Reduction in the Mineral Content of Food Crops?" Dept of Soil Science, University of Wisconsin, Madison, USA.
(b) Mineral Depletion of the Soil and the Importance of Minerals for Man's Longevity, Senate Document No. 264, 1936.

Dangers in Pregnancy

Ironically, a number of the major dangers during pregnancy can involve the dentist, some of which are described below.

X-rays and Pregnancy

X-rays are extremely high energy microwaves and are a potent source of change to the cell and genetic structure of any living organism

It is because of dental X-rays that dentists must know about a patient's pregnancy. The dangers of X-rays during pregnancy have long been a basic part of dental training, and although dental doses are tiny in comparison to those used on the body generally, they should not be taken on pregnant mums.

In a similar situation, I wonder if any research has been done on the effects microwave ovens can have on a developing child. The effects, for instance, of visual display units (VDUs—computer screens) on workers have often been highlighted.[50] Headaches and aching eyes were the least of these. More research is definitely needed in this field because environmentally we are surrounded by a variety of electromagnetic waves, which could, like X-rays, affect genetics as well as growing structures.

Mercury (Hg)

The placenta, previously thought of as a barrier to prevent toxic substances reaching the baby, is in reality a membrane through which both good and bad substances of all sorts can pass. One of the big "baddies" is mercury, a major constituent (50 percent) of the amalgam used in dental amalgam fillings. Mercury is undeniably a poisonous element, the third most toxic on this planet. Any

---

50   VDU Work and Hazards to Health, Copyright 1993, London Hazards Centre, 213 Haverstock Hill, London NW3 4QP, UK.

amalgam filling work can release mercury vapor, which, however slight, can concentrate in the fetus.

Given that we know mercury can cause problems, even if it's in the smallest amounts (there are no safe lower limits), we want to reduce that amount to the barest minimum. The only answer is not to disturb amalgam fillings at all during pregnancy and during lactation, as mercury can pass into breast milk as well. It is a temptation for a mother and for a dentist to get old or new filling work done at the same time as the gum problem is being sorted out, but it is placing baby at great risk. Dentists should do routine examinations, scaling, give nutritional advice and advice on cleaning—the latter a major factor in controlling gum problems—but avoid fillings if possible. In Great Britain, the disturbance and placement of amalgam fillings during pregnancy has been effectively banned under the NHS—a good move.

Lead (Pb)

Another heavy metal hazard is lead, which has been shown to concentrate, like mercury, in the fetus. I feel that pregnant women ought to minimize traveling in cars while there is still any chance of lead (or lead substitutes such as MTBE) in gasoline.[51] Any mother who lives near a major road or in the center of an industrial town or city should be aware of the possible effects of pollution upon her unborn child. This is where an organization like Foresight can play such an important part, doing tests to check levels of toxins in general. The hair analysis is particularly effective because although the hair is dead, it was formed from general body tissues and can show three months of accumulation, whether vitamin, mineral, or toxin. This is an effective test to perform, as it is primarily noninvasive, does not interfere with the body, and is also uniquely informative.

Lead and other toxins can also be taken in through the skin as well as the nose and mouth. Hands should be washed well before preparing food; fruit and vegetables bought or grown in industrial

---

51 Lead TetraEthyl and MTBE, Simon Cotton, Uppingham School, Rutland, UK.

areas should be washed well. All chemicals that might be inhaled, and these include spirit-based paints and lots of gardening products, should be completely avoided during pregnancy. Mercury is still used as a pesticide/fungicide,[52] which is another good reason to buy organic.

Pharmaceutical Drugs

I would emphasize again that, whenever possible, drugs should be avoided during pregnancy; indeed, ever since the thalidomide tragedy,[53] the medical profession and the public have been all too aware of the effects drugs can have on the fetus. As mentioned in the section on preconceptual care, any drug taking for a long-term condition will have been discussed previously with a doctor and possibly modified. It's not only oral drugs that can harm, but also many creams or ointments for external use. Those creams for eczema, for example, are potentially hazardous[54] if used or administered by an expectant mother.

Tetracycline[55] (an antibiotic) can have a dramatic effect on calcifying teeth and causing severe discoloration. All patent remedies for colds, indigestion, nausea, and other minor ailments should also be avoided. Again, if in doubt, don't!

---

52 (a) Natural Resources Conservation Service (USA), Conservation Practice Standard, Pesticide Risk Mitigator, Code 596.
   (b) Using EHP Biologic Markers in Blood to Assess Exposure to Multiple Environmental Chemicals for Inner-City Children Aged 3–6 years.
   (c) EHP Environmental Health Perspectives, Ken Sexton et al:
   (i) University of Texas, School of Public Health, Texas, USA
   (ii) University of Minnesota, School of Public Health
   (iii) Centres of Disease Control and Prevention, Allanton, Georgia,. USA, May 16 2005.
53 Thalidomide: 40 Years On, BBC News, UK—http://news.bbc.co.uk/1/hi/uk/2031459.stm
54 (a) Eczema—A Topic Clinical Summary (NHS)
   (b) Patient Information Leaflet (NHS)
   (c) GSK Safety Data Sheet for Eumovate Cream, 17 March 2009.
55 http://absoluteacneinfo.com/tetracycline/—Side Effects Relating to Tetracycline

Coffee (yes, including decaffeinated), tea, cocoa, chocolate, and cola drinks all contain the drug caffeine, and they should be cut out of the maternal diet. Herbal teas and pure juices could be substituted. Tea also contains fluoride, which can have an effect on the bones and teeth of the growing child. Conscientious mothers often believe that by taking fluoride tablets during pregnancy, they are helping their baby's teeth. There is in fact no conclusive proof that this does help, or indeed does harm, but as fluoride interferes with calcium metabolism, we do not know the effects of extra fluoride on growing teeth and bones. As an example, some mothers drink up to twenty cups of tea a day. If they are also using fluoridated water, and perhaps taking tablets, they could be ingesting far too much fluoride, which could have a deleterious effect on their babies.

Smoking

Smoking cigarettes is a major source of the toxic metal cadmium and of the drug nicotine. Smoking by the mother will increase the blood levels of carbon monoxide in the bloodstream of the smoking mother, and this will pass into the baby's bloodstream. This can starve it of oxygen, resulting in poor development, a condition known as "Fetal Origins of Disease."[56] Babies born to smoking mothers may appear similar to a baby born a month prematurely. Poor body growths as well as poor intellectual growth are the results. Smoking is a major evil for unborn children, and it must be avoided at all costs. It is reassuring that all medical authorities concur that smoking is bad for you and your growing baby.

Alcohol

Any amount of alcohol may harm a baby in the womb, and the baby is particularly vulnerable to such damage in the first eight to twelve weeks of development, another pointer to the necessity of cutting it out before conception to allow for the first few weeks

---

56   Bergen, H. "Exposure to Smoke during Development: Foetal Programming of Adult Disease," Dept of Human Anatomy and Cell Science, University of Manitoba, 2006.

of uncertainty as to whether conception has taken place. Alcohol will pass through the placenta, and in later months, it is believed,[57] affect the development of the fetal brain, resulting in fetal alcohol syndrome (FAS).

Food Additives

Additives are the bane of the modern diet—every holistic practitioner battles against these—and every other medical practitioner should. For commercial reasons—for ease of manufacture, for customer temptation, for a longer shelf life—colorings, antioxidants, flavorings, preservatives, and so on, are added to foods. Few are nutrients; indeed, not many do us any good. Some even deprive the foods of what basic nutritional value they have. If we are beginning to realize that they can cause harm to grown bodies, the effect that they could have on growing bodies is too disturbing to contemplate.

In Britain, we seem to have been slower in cutting out many of these additives, thus many of the foods on sale here are looked upon as unsafe, and even poisonous, in other countries. You should avoid processed or refined foods whenever possible, which is a piece of advice that has cropped up many times before. Baking an organic potato in the oven is just as simple, if more lengthy than adding water to dried potato granules, and preparing a green vegetable and steaming it for a few minutes takes no more time or energy than opening a pack or a can, and it is so much healthier.

Not enough is currently known about the effects of additives on the body in general, or on the developing fetus. To eliminate all the risks, remove all foods containing additives. Go organic!

A little known fact: many of the toxins stored by the expectant mum are "dumped" into the fetus[58]!

---

57   Alcohol Alert—National Institute on Alcohol Abuse and Alcoholism, NIAAA, PO Box 10686, Rockville, MD 20849-0686, USA
58   (a) Vanderbilt University, Pregnancy and Fish (Do We Really Have To Give Up?), Courtney Mijel, 11 12 2005.

Brian Halvorsen, BDS, LDS RCS

Postnatal Care

Right from the moment the new baby draws breath, there are many dental significances. And the first one, literally, involves that first breath. The mouth, as indeed the body, generally nurtures a vast variety of bacteria, some of it benign and some not nearly so pleasant. We can assume that at the moment of birth, the baby's mouth is free of bacteria. As soon as the baby leaves the womb and breathes in, it will absorb the ambient bacteria and many other viruses and yeasts existing in the air on the baby's parents' skin, even in the supposedly sterile delivery room. These bacteria will form the basis of the baby's own unique oral environment, and they can dictate whether they might ultimately be vulnerable to tooth decay and gum disease. So are the aforementioned conditions hereditary? Partly, but other factors have an important role.

However, less speculatively, at birth the baby's toothless gums will be holding within them some forty-four teeth, consisting of twenty baby, or deciduous, teeth, together with the germs of twenty-four of the permanent teeth. At this stage, all are at some vital stage of development. If the birth is prolonged[59] and disrupts the growth of the baby, this can show up on the permanent teeth when they start to erupt five to eight years later. If the tooth or teeth were being calcified at the time of birth, then there would be signs of this with the neonatal line, sometimes only visible to the professional's eyes or sometimes quite obvious, especially as a horizontal shadow or defect in the front teeth.

Other factors that could disturb the teeth at birth include prematurity and hemolytic anemia (jaundice). A premature baby may be born without reserves of certain vital minerals, such as calcium and iron, that can affect the teeth. Indeed, the prematurity may have been caused to some extent by some deficiency in the normal growth of the child. Babies who are born too soon will probably have to

---

(b) Silicon Valley Toxics Coalition (SVTC), http://www.etoxics.org/site/PageServer?pagename=svtc_toxics_in_electronics

59 Skinner, M; Dupras T. "Variation in Birth Timing and Location of the Neonatal Line in Human Enamel," Simon Frazer University, British Columbia, Canada; School of Human Biology, University of Guelph, Ontario, Canada, 1992–93

be kept in incubation, given drips, fed artificially, etc., and all this trauma could affect the tooth formation that will be going on at this time. A baby born with jaundice, due to an incompatibility of the cells of baby and mother, can lead to discoloration of the teeth that are being formed at that time.[60]

Breastfeeding

A mother who breastfeeds her baby is giving it the best possible start in life. Provided the mother is continuing the good, sensible, and nourishing diet she ate while the baby was growing in her womb, her milk is perfectly formulated for the baby. It contains all the protein, vitamins, calcium and other minerals in the right proportions for the baby's total and correct nutrition, and manufacturers cannot improve on it. The colostrum that comes through in the first few days, a sticky yellow substance which precedes the milk proper, contains many antibodies from the mother that will protect the baby from a number of the infections and illnesses that could cause bodily and dental problems. It is also very high in vitamin A, which is important for teeth. Enzymes in unheated milk, breast milk, help with hardening of the bones and teeth. The protein molecules in breast milk are considerably smaller than those contained in cows' milk, and therefore protein and calcium are absorbed much more successfully. Altogether, it has been said that breast milk can mean fewer infections, fewer allergic diseases, less coeliac disease, fewer crib deaths, and less future obesity and heart disease.[61]

Holistically, and from a nutritional point of view, I would recommend breastfeeding only, and for at least four months. However, it is undeniable that some mothers just cannot breastfeed, whether because of illness or merely because they cannot seem to produce enough milk. Sometimes breastfeeding is avoided because of social inconvenience. In all cases, if possible, I would hope that mothers would persevere, and be encouraged to persevere, for in some

---

60 Cheng K., "Potential Problems with Baby teeth
    Source; www.yourtotalhealth.ivillage.com
61 Williams, Rebecca. "Breastfeeding Best Bet for Babies." FDA, US Food and Drug Administration, Oct 1995.

maternity hospitals, if there is difficulty, a baby is immediately put on the bottle and on formula cows' milk. Even if breastfeeding cannot be continued, the mother should at least give the baby the colostrum of the first five days or so, as it is so rich in protective factors.

The phrase that nutritionists quote in this context is: "Mother's milk is perfect for babies; cows' milk is perfect for calves." Cows' milk, however, modified for milk powders, is much more concentrated in almost everything, which is not so surprising when you consider that a calf will grow from its birth weight to about five or six hundred pounds (225–270 kilograms) in its first year!

Although some milk formulas are fairly well balanced, and are being improved all the time, they are not the natural food for babies. Millions of babies appear to thrive on them, of course, but I would rather see a return to the most natural form of baby feeding, that from the breast.

The other major advantage of breastfeeding your baby is that it gives a better jaw and mouth development. Many dentists and dental specialists[62] have reported that they see fewer problems of jaw and tooth development in breastfed babies. In a survey of some five hundred children with jaw problems requiring orthodontic work, only two had been breastfed! The principal cause is thought to be the unnatural action of the muscles of the mouth and tongue that are brought into play when a baby sucks from a bottle. Often, teat holes on a bottle are too large, which means that the milk can gush down a baby's throat, depriving him or her of the most basic desire: to suck.

Dr. B Palmer, DDS, concludes, "Breastfeeding reduces the risk of the malocclusions ('bite relationships') that can put an individual at risk for obstructive sleep apnea (OSA). Since OSA can lead to many

---

62 (a) Barnetson, B. "Breast-feeding, Bottles and Pacifiers: The Importance of Jaw Development on Reducing Ear Infections." Families for Natural Living (FNL)—http://www.familiesfornaturalliving.org/ONSITE/render.php
(b) Bahr, D. "Oral Motor Assessment and Treatment." Diane Bahr of Ages and Stages®, LLC, March 2003,http://oral-motor.com/_wsn/page11.html

health problems, it can be concluded that breastfeeding is critical for the future health of our children.[63]"

Sucking from a bottle is easier than from the breast, which is a contributory factor. As sucking is such a natural instinct, and the nipple is the natural thing to suck upon, any other action, even such as sucking on the bottle teat, could justifiably be termed abnormal. Bottle-fed babies can exhibit several types of malocclusion or crookedness of the teeth, which will probably require orthodontic treatment in the future. New teats that imitate the action of the nipple have been developed, and this, it is hoped, will reduce this tendency to malocclusion in bottle-fed babies.

The last, and certainly not the least, advantage of feeding from the breast is the undoubted greater intimacy between mother and child. Although babies who are bottle-fed are held in the same position, and will probably receive as many cuddles and kisses, a closer relationship does seem to develop in breastfeeding. It is difficult to prove in any scientific way, but perhaps it is because a breastfed baby who cries will be picked up, comforted, and probably fed as well. A bottle-fed baby may have to wait for that feeding comfort until the correct feeding time, or at least until the bottle is prepared. I am sure that the physical contact between mother and baby has deep long-term physiological benefits for the growing child.

Maternal Diet during Lactation

As during pregnancy, the need for essential nutrients is higher, and milk production can drain a breastfeeding mother as much as can the demands of the growing baby in the womb. A good diet will ensure that the milk is of good quality and that the mother's health is maintained. Foods rich in B vitamins[64] will help counteract tiredness and stress. Small, frequent meals might keep your metabolism going, even aiding in weight loss, and be more palatable than three larger ones (however, remember to brush your teeth well afterward). The

---

63   www.brianpalmerdds.com, Brian Palmer, DDS, For Better Health.
64   Rutherford, D. "Sources of Vitamins." http://www.netdoctor.co.uk/menshealth/wellbeing/vitamins_minerals/vitamin.htm

mother should increase her daily liquid intake while breastfeeding to ensure a good milk supply.

Dental work should still be avoided because of the mercury dangers; alcohol and many drugs such as aspirin, laxatives, sedatives, etc., can enter the breast milk. Smoking can also reduce the milk supply, and antibiotics, particularly tetracycline, can affect the baby, while returning to the contraceptive pill[65] can also reduce milk supply slightly.

If the mother is careful at this stage in every way, and if she is well fed and the baby is well fed too as a result, the likelihood of contracting any infection is substantially reduced. It is in these first few months that many babies develop the colds, snuffles, and feverish illnesses that can have an effect on the teeth. There is no doubt that there is a relationship between diet and a good resistance to disease, whether bodily or dentally.

Teething

Despite all the risks and insults—biochemical, dietary, and genetic— that can afflict a new baby, it is quite a tribute to the composition of human beings that most babies are born normally, grow normally, and their teeth grow relatively normally as well. Baby teeth seem to be the least affected by growth anomalies.

The charts below show the approximate order and timing of the appearance of the baby, or deciduous, teeth. However, the timing is only a rough guide, as many babies can remain toothless until they are at least one year old! The timing mechanisms are part of the baby's own individual blueprint, perhaps part of a pattern that it has inherited, and the teeth will come through when they are ready. Teething usually starts, though, when the baby is about six months, and all the deciduous teeth are usually through by the age of two and a half years (the chart also shows the chronology of eruption of root and crown completion and calcification).

---

65 Brown, S. "Can I Use Birth Control Pills While Breastfeeding?" About. com http://babyparenting.about.com/cs/breastfeeding/f/bcnursing.htm

Great Teeth for Life

Chronology of the Deciduous Teeth

Tooth	Initial Calcification	Completion of Crown	Eruption	Completion of Roots
Upper first incisor	3–4 months in utero	4 months	7½ months	1½–2 years
Lower first incisor	4½ months in utero	4 months	6½ months	1½–2 years
Upper second incisor	4½ months in utero	5 months	8 months	1½–2 years
Lower second incisor	4½ months in utero	4½ months	7 months	1½–2 years
Upper canine	5 months in utero	9 months	16–20 months	2½–3 years
Lower canine	5 months in utero	9 months	16–20 months	2½–3 years
Upper first molar	5 months in utero	6 months	12–16 months	2½–3 years
Lower first molar	5 months in utero	6 months	12–16 months	2½–3 years
Upper second molar	6 months in utero	10–12 months	1¾–2½ years	3 years
Lower second molar	6 months in utero	10–12 months	1¾–2½ years	3 years

Adapted from a chart based on the work of Logan and Kröfeld, reproduced in Dental Morphology by G. C. Van Beek BDS(Brist), (Wright Pub)[66]

Chronology of the Permanent Teeth

Tooth	Initial Calcification	Completion of Crown	Eruption	Completion of Roots
Upper first incisor	3–4 months	4–5 years	7–8 years	10 years
Lower first incisor	3–4 months	4–5 years	6–7 years	9 years
Upper second incisor	10–12 months	4–5 years	8–9 years	11 years
Lower second incisor	3–4 months	4–5 years	7–8 years	10 years
Upper canine	4–5 months	6–7 years	11–12 years	13–15 years
Lower canine	4–5 months	6–7 years	9–10 years	12–14 years
Upper first premolar	1½–2 years	5–6years	10–11 years	12–13 years
Lower first premolar	1¾–2 years	5–6years	10–12 years	12–13 years
Upper second premolar	2–2½ years	6–7 years	10–12 years	12–14 years
Lower second premolar	2¼–2½	6–7 years	11–12 years	13–14 years
Upper first molar	Birth or slightly before	2½–3 years	6–7 years	9–10 years
Lower first molar	Birth or slightly before	2½–3 years	6–7 years	9–10 years
Upper second molar	2½–3 years	7–8 years	12–13 years	14–16 years
Lower second molar	2½–3 years	7–8 years	12–13 years	14–15 years
Upper third molar	7–9 years	12–16 years	17–21years	18–25 years
Lower third molar	8–10 years	12–16 years	17–21 years	18–25 years

Adapted from a chart based on the work of Logan and Kröfeld, reproduced in Dental Morphology by G. C. Van Beek BDS(Brist), (Wright Pub)

The baby is born with the baby teeth already formed in the gums. No one quite knows what causes them to erupt, but it may be that

---

66   http://www.amazon.co.uk/Dental-Morphology-Van-Beek-Brist/dp/0723606668/ref=sr_1_1?ie=UTF8&s=books&qid=1244120890&sr=8-1

the periodontal fibers grow and stretch, pushing the teeth through the gums. However, we do know that the teething process can be painful to the baby—and to the parents!

The first signs of teething may be reddish gums, a bump showing on the gums, dribbling, and red patches on the cheek. All this affects some babies, but not all. It is an uncomfortable time for the gums, not surprising, with the hardest substance in the body pushing through them.

To ease this, I cannot recommend any of the topical reliefs that you rub on the baby's gums. They are not particularly effective, and you will also be introducing the baby to drugs and chemicals of which we do not know the long-term effects. Some of the gels and powders (one brand used to contain mercury) are likely to be swallowed. The same applies to the pain-relieving syrups, which are swallowed, and many of them are packed with sugar, which is bad both dentally and from the point of view that you are perhaps familiarizing a baby with a sweet taste.

Cuddles and comfort would be a major relieving factor, with a clean finger perhaps rubbed onto the sore gum. At least this will assure an irritable baby that you're aware of the problem and that you care. Cold teething rings or hard chewing sticks can help, but a ring should only be fridge cold (not freezer cold which can "burn" the gums and lips). Anything the baby has put in the mouth must be scrupulously clean and safe (large enough so that it cannot be swallowed and strong enough that no part can fracture off).

Teething is often associated with red bottoms or an increase in nappy rash. Teething isn't an infection, but it is an inflammation of sorts, and what is happening in the mouth can and does seem to "echo" itself on the baby's bottom! Scrupulous cleaning and frequent nappy changing will help prevent the problem from becoming worse.

Teething is used as a convenient scapegoat for almost everything. It is blamed for irritability, diarrhea, fevers, sickness, and loss of appetite. In reality, however, none of these are related at all to teething, except perhaps the latter, and if a baby does seem to go off its food, the doctor may need to be consulted. Babies do get grizzly with the discomforts of teething, but they should still be hungry, should still need food, their most basic requirement.

As soon as the baby teeth erupt, they must be kept clean. Most experts advise[67] the mother to clean around the tooth or teeth and gums with a small piece of clean gauze or a cotton-wool bud.

Some suggest using a little toothpaste on a gauze or cloth, but I would not advise this, as toothpastes, even "natural" ones, are quite chemically strong, and some is likely to be swallowed

It is not necessarily the toothpaste that cleans anyway; it is the massage and rubbing. A soft toothbrush can be used later, perhaps with the merest suggestion of toothpaste, which will help accustom the child to brushing and indeed, when he or she is allowed to hold and use the brush itself, it can become a pleasurable game.

Moving on from Breast Milk Alone

Breastfeeding should be carried on as long as possible, and unless there is a good reason for it, mothers shouldn't feel that there is a great rush to move their babies on to mixed feeding. Recently, there was a lot of pressure on parents to start this process early, within the first three months (often for commercial, and occasionally for medical, reasons). Breast milk is all that is needed for at least the first four months, and it can be carried on for longer while weaning. A baby introduced to foods other than milk will suck less at the breast. The breasts will therefore get less stimulation and will produce less milk; and the baby will ultimately not get enough milk, forcing a change to solids. Care must be taken that this does not occur too early.

This has both a nutritional significance, as milk is the optimum food for growth at this stage, and a developmental significance: the lack of sucking will also affect the jaws. In addition, a baby's digestive system is not capable of absorbing foods more complex than milk until at least three months old.

---

67 American Academy of Pediatric Dentistry, Dental Care for Your Baby, http://www.aapd.org/publications/brochures/babycare.asp

Often a mother can feel instinctively when her baby is ready to start solids, i.e., something other than milk. If baby seems restless and hungry before four months, he should be allowed to suckle longer at each feeding, or he could be fed more frequently throughout the day. Only in exceptional cases should this be read as the signal that he wants to move on to other foods, but if after four months he shows the same signs, he may be ready.

Another sign can be when the birth weight has doubled, or when weight increase has slowed down considerably. By about six months old, however, the baby often does need more nutrients than milk alone can supply, although milk from the breast can and should still remain a valuable part of the diet for as long as the mother wishes to continue feeding.

Check carefully after each new introduction of food to see that it does not have an adverse effect—causing diarrhea, for example—and try only one food at a time, so that if there is a reaction, the food can be pinpointed accurately and immediately assessed for sensitivities. Rejecting the food in question may not necessarily mean that the baby has an allergy—it may mean that he is just not ready yet.

Juices

The first things to try are juices, from about four to five months, and therefore perhaps one of the first investments for your baby's health ought to be a juice extractor. Don't just think of the citrus fruits with their high content of vitamin C. Cauliflower, cabbage, turnip, and green beans also contain vitamin C in good quantities, as well as a variety of other nutrients such as calcium.

Carrots, the traditional "first" vegetable for babies, contain a digestible form of calcium as well as vitamin A, and they can easily be liquidized. Most of the vitamins from vegetables and fruit are contained near the skin, but all have to be peeled or at least washed and scraped because the skin is the fibrous part of the plant. The baby's digestive system could not cope with this, however, and another consideration is that the vegetable or fruit might have been sprayed (do try to buy organic and unsprayed products at all times).

All juices must be diluted with cooled, boiled filtered water, as their nutrients are too concentrated at this stage. Start with one teaspoon a day. Just because a baby seems to like carrot juice, for example, don't necessarily give it to him daily for the next week. This may bore the baby, and it's fun for them and for you to try a wide variety of tastes, as long as basic precautions are taken. Try peach or mango, apple or tomato (sieve to remove any skin or seeds). Do be wary, though, for some citrus fruits and strawberries can trigger allergies, so they should perhaps be considered for a later stage. When you start experimenting with juices, you can be very inventive, and there are many alternatives.

If you cannot afford to buy a juice extractor, chopped vegetables can be puréed with some cooled boiled water in an electric blender or food processor. When puréed, strain through a fine mesh metal sieve to retain any fibrous material. Do not heat juices, as this will destroy many of the vitamins.

The one thing to avoid is commercial fruit juice, especially those made with babies in mind, because they can be made with a sweet syrup base. Stick to pure, unadulterated fruit and vegetable juices with no additives or preservatives. I'm not even entirely happy about carton juices, which are designated pure and may indeed have no additives or preservatives, but they have been conditioned or heated, which detracts, I think, from their nutritional value, although they are acceptable to use as a standby.

Purées

The next phase of mixed infant feeding is purées, which require little or no chewing. These should be introduced slowly, with only one teaspoon being offered at one meal (at lunchtime, for example, when the baby is not as hungry as in the morning). The texture should be fairly wet and soft at first, thinned down with breast milk, filtered water, or water that has been boiled and cooled.

All the different baby books[68] available give plenty of ideas for the best foods to serve as purées, and those to avoid. Things like ripe bananas, carrots, apples, and pears are good first foods. Cooking, of course, takes away some of the vitamins, but apples and carrots do have to be lightly cooked before mashing or puréeing. A food offered at body temperature instead of cold will probably be accepted more easily anyway; perhaps heat slightly so that the chill is taken off. Another excellent fruit, rich in vitamin E and unsaturated fatty acids, is the avocado pear, which mashes down easily like banana.

Many experts[69] say that a cereal is a good first purée type food, but beware, as there is a small possibility of celiac disease (gluten allergy) from wheat cereals such as wholemeal porridge and semolina, etc. Other wholegrain cereals could be too high[70] in fiber for a baby. These could have a locking-up effect on the calcium as well as zinc and magnesium. Remember to avoid calcium-robbing foods such as rhubarb and spinach. Many baby cereals have added vitamins, which sounds beneficial, but along with all the vitamins in the natural food, plus possible supplements, this could be creating an imbalance. One of the better cereals in terms of allergies, for instance, is baby rice, but it too has had various things added to it, such as vitamins and minerals. These "artificial" additives can unbalance the natural ratios of vitamins found in nature, and I would prefer to see a more natural vitamin intake using fresh fruits and vegetables only.

In the early 1980s, companies in West Germany produced organic baby foods. Now a huge variety of organic baby foods and recipes

68 (a) Your Feeding Questions Answered by Annabel Karmel, http://www.amazon.co.uk/Feeding-Questions-Answered-Annabel-Karmel/dp/140533536X/ref=sr_1_1?ie=UTF8&s=books&qid=1244121297&sr=8-1
(b) Recipes for Babies, Healthy, Organic, Pure, Nutritious, http://www.organix.com/
(c) The Baby's Table, Brenda Bradshaw and Lauren Bramley, Random House, Canada
69 When Should You Start Feeding Cereal to Your Baby? By Sue Gilbert, MS, http://parenting.ivillage.com/baby/bnutrition/0,,3vp7,00.html
70 Nutrition for Children and for Infants, Medic8 Family Health Guide, www.medic8.com/healthguide/

is available. Many of the preprepared baby foods sold in jars and cans in the United Kingdom, however, still have coloring, sugars, and salts added, and although they are getting better, they should only be used in emergencies. It is appropriate to mention here, too, that mothers should always look at the labels of baby foods if they must buy them. It will be a salutary lesson to see how much is added—or how much the foods are modified—and it must always be remembered that the ingredients are listed in diminishing quantity order. If water is first, it means that there is more water than anything else!

One of the best foods at this stage must be the sprout of seeds and pulses. Many plants can be sprouted: soya beans, chickpeas, fenugreek seeds, lentils, buckwheat, and the sprouts that enrich so many Chinese dishes, those of the Mung bean. Sprouts are easy to grow at home and are inexpensive. One pound (450 grams) of seeds or beans can yield seven to ten pounds (3-4.5 kilograms) of sprouts! They are completely free of allergens and pollutants, and they are rich in nutrients for everyone, particularly babies. They contain virtually the whole range of vitamins and easily digestible protein.

During the sprouting process, the proteins inside the seed or pulse are converted to amino acids, which are the constituents of protein. Therefore, the actual sprouting process itself has already undertaken part of the digestive process. In order to visualize more clearly the nutrients that are locked up and then released by sprouting, consider the simple sunflower seed. Think of the size of the seed and then the size of the plant. All the potential for that growth is contained within one tiny seed!

The best seed for babies is probably alfalfa, the smallest seed to sprout. Put a handful of seeds in a large, clean glass jar and cover with water. Leave to soak for an hour or so and then cover the top of the jar with muslin or a piece of J Cloth secured with an elastic band. Drain the water away through the cloth and put the jar into a dry, dark place. Repeat the soaking and draining procedure once a day and the sprouts should be ready in about three to four days. When ready, remove from the jar and place them in a bowl of cold water. Stir around to free the husks, the fibrous part, which should float to the surface and can be tipped away. Cut away any remaining husks and purée the root and the sprout, moistening them with a little cooled boiled water or breast milk.

Solid Foods

The chewing reflex is always present, and as the baby gets older and eats more, the digestive system becomes more sophisticated and can cope with rougher, thicker textures, which could more justifiably be termed "solid" foods.[71] Many babies are put on solid foods far too quickly because it is thought they need to get their jaws working properly. Their jaws are already working quite adequately, and a new choice and texture of foods is only relevant from the point of view that the baby has an increased choice of nutrients.

When moving on from purées, do so gradually. Use one teaspoon of diced foods to half a cup of puréed foods to get a texture that will be acceptable. The diced foods must be soft—no fibrous meat at this stage—for the gum will be doing most of the chewing work. Keep an eye on how the foods are being digested. If the baby is spitting them out, getting tummy pains, or the food is passing through in chunks, the baby may not be quite ready for this texture stage. The digestive system may not be mature, or the baby isn't managing to chew the food enough in the mouth to start the digestive process.

Never forget about finger foods, which are good for gums and teething. In the earlier stages, there are dangers of pieces flaking off some finger foods and causing the baby to choke. But most finger foods will massage gums, clean tiny teeth once they erupt, and feed the baby well at the same time. Try peeled, quartered, and cored apples, peeled raw carrots, fingers of peeled cucumber or prepared vegetables, and baked crusts of wholemeal bread.

At some time within this first year, usually at about eight months, many babies are weaned off the breast (or the bottle), and are put on cows' milk. I have already mentioned my misgivings about cows' milk for young babies. I feel that the emphasis so many child

---

71   (a)   http://www.babycenter.com/0_introducing-solid-foods_113.bc
     (b)   http://www.eatwell.gov.uk/agesandstages/baby/weaning/   Food Standards Agency, Eat Well, Be Well

nutritionists place on the milk content of a child's diet is perhaps overstated. It is the calcium and vitamins and minerals that are considered vital, but all of these can come from a good sensible whole food diet, thus cutting out the necessity for a large intake of milk, even if the milk and milk products are organic!

Some may consider this revolutionary, but cows' milk does contain sodium in excess; it does have protein in larger, more indigestible molecules; and it may well contain hormones, antibiotics, and stabilizers. It is worth consulting your pediatrician for alternatives to dairy products if necessary.

The basic point is that once the baby is off the breast or bottle, it is not entirely necessary for her to continue drinking milk. If the baby is on a good diet, with lots of sprouts, vegetable, and fruit purées, etc., she will be getting enough calcium and other essentials.

One of the milk products of which I do approve is yogurt, and this can be useful from the earliest mixed feeding stages onwards. For those who feel I may be contradicting the norm, flying in the face of accepted thinking, yogurt is, of course, milk, but it is milk that is converted into a much more soluble form of calcium by the yogurt bacteria. It should be live and natural, and it is best made at home from organic milk.

Fruit can be added to it for a change, and that is far more nourishing and satisfactory than commercial fruit yogurts, which can have up to one tablespoon of sugar in them! Again, organic yogurts and milk products are available in most supermarkets in Europe. The transition from breast milk to no milk, if you choose to do this, should be slow, however, and yogurt will be a good substitute along with the other infant foods already mentioned above.

For those who eat meat, it should be introduced in small amounts at first, and it should always be obtained from trustworthy sources, if possible, to ensure that no growth promoters or hormones have been used to make the animals put on weight. Butchery and hanging should have been carried out in the old traditional ways, which will give the best flavor and quality. Many holistic and whole food nutritionists are against meat in general, and they advocate alternative protein sources, but I believe meat can be acceptable, provided it is in smallish quantities, as it is undoubtedly rich in good proteins for babies, and it contains many of the fats that they need.

Try to avoid the richer meats such as beef, lamb, and pork, serving poultry instead. Fish is an equally good source of protein and other essentials, while liver is also nutritious, providing vitamin K and iron. Of course, all foods should be organically sourced and consumed in well-balanced quantities.

When cooking for the family and the baby, remember that a baby needn't grow up with a yearning or taste for seasoned foods. Their taste buds do not crave sugar or salt, so there is no need to introduce baby to them. When cooking, do not use salt. Add salt to food at the table.

A basic dietary rule is that foods in general should be as natural and as lightly cooked as possible.

Eating with the Family

Once the baby has all the baby teeth and is eating and enjoying a wide range of good foods, he will be able to join in with family meals. In fact, the earlier he can do this the better, for he can learn that eating in company is enjoyable, which can help prevent eating problems later. And, of course, it's all part of the learning process.

Many conscientious parents do tend to feed their baby the best possible foods, preparing them with the utmost care, whilst carrying on the same bad dietary habits themselves. There's a lot to be said for the whole family changing its eating habits at this stage, or even earlier, so that the baby's ultimate health, and that of the rest of the family, can be ensured.

Children from about two years onward have different growth phases and differing appetites, and many eating problems occur at this age. Parental example is a major influence. If you eat and enjoy your lightly cooked greens, the chances are the baby will too, but any apparent reluctance to do so may just be that the baby isn't hungry or because he's going through a quiescent period of growth.

Just because a baby or child won't eat, don't cram him full of sugars because you think that anything—a favorite pudding, for example—is better than nothing. In general, puddings aren't good nutritionally, but if you have only yogurt or fruit available, these could be light and enjoyable, and fruit will quench the thirst as well as feed.

Deciduous Teeth and the Dentist

Holistic dentists would like to be involved with children's teeth right from the beginning, and obviously this depends to a large extent on the parent and his or her relationship with the dentist. We would hope, as already mentioned, to have given advice before conception and during pregnancy, but often it happens that a mother gets so involved after having the baby, and there is a quite natural reluctance to bring a screaming baby into the surgery, so she may not consult the dentist again at least for twelve months!

This lost time as far as her own dental health is concerned could be alarming, but it is also a time when the dentist could be contributing a great deal to the future dental health of her child.

He can help with teething problems, continue the dietary advice, and become aware of any potential problems as the child's teeth develop. When a new parent comes to the dentist for a checkup or treatment at regular intervals, the child should be brought along too.

This can alleviate all sorts of worries on all sides. The baby and toddler will gradually become accustomed to the man in the white coat and will become familiar with the smells of a dental office. The parents will also be able to gain reassurance in all aspects of their child's teeth that might be worrying them.

Deciduous Abnormalities

Baby teeth usually grow without any problems. The most common worry is about timing. If a neighbor's baby has all its front teeth, and yours is still grinning toothlessly, don't think that your baby is backward; teeth just take their own time.

If a parent is worried about the position of a child's teeth as they erupt—if they don't sit centrally on the gum ridge, for example—the dentist can also reassure the patient. This is where the action of the lips and the tongue will come into play. Even if the baby's teeth are not in the correct position when they erupt, the lips, tongue, and cheeks will soon push them into a nice arc.

It is also important that the dentist can look at the jaw size and shape, and the spacing of the teeth, of a baby and child. It is not unusual, for instance, that the upper jaw protrudes more than the lower jaw in baby dentition. This does not necessarily mean that they will retain this appearance in the permanent teeth, although genetics will play a part. If nutrition has been good throughout pregnancy and thereafter, the jaw will be given the potential to be wide, allowing good spacing between the teeth. Again, genetic factors should be considered; a father or mother who has had crowded baby teeth and then required orthodontic extractions or treatment on his or her permanent teeth may have passed this on to their child.

Crowded baby teeth may mean crowded permanent teeth, and this needs careful monitoring, as crowding increases the vulnerability to tooth decay and gum disease. Parents should be given detailed advice from the dentist on diet so that foods that can cause decay, like sugars and refined carbohydrates, can be assiduously avoided. Advice on tooth brushing and oral hygiene can be given to Mom and Dad, as they are responsible for baby's dental health.

Tooth Decay and Deciduous Teeth

It is vital that baby teeth are looked after well, and it is the sole responsibility of the parent to monitor diet and cleaning for at least the entire deciduous period, and indeed throughout the complete period of mixed dentition, which is up to about the age of nine or ten.

Sugars and sweet eating should always be discouraged. Children's drinks, too, although often advertised as being full of vitamin C, are so full of sugar that any benefits are completely nullified. Pure fruit or vegetable juices, heavily diluted sugar-free juices, or just plain water are all that are needed, and if a child is eating a good, nourishing whole food diet, he or she won't be all that thirsty. Coating a baby's dummy, or pacifier, with a syrupy drink or honey is bad news. It may temporarily placate a screaming baby or toddler, but the ensuing traumas when tooth decay occurs, and the dental treatment that will follow, far outweigh any such short-lived peace.

A child with tooth decay will have to go to the dentist for treatment, and he may have to undergo drilling, filling, fear, and discomfort. No dentist wishes to inflict this upon anyone, especially a toddler.

A child of three or four will not have the patience to sit in a dental chair for longer than a few minutes, so treatment can often be difficult. Any discomfort experienced at this stage could have a permanent effect on the child and her perception of the dentist in years to come. Dentists, too, experience problems when they encounter tooth decay in baby teeth. They would like to build up a relationship with their patients in an advisory, caring sense, discussing such problems as crowding and staining. Dentists do not want to have to drill and fill or extract teeth to perform what is in effect destructive treatment, and to treat a disease that could have been prevented.

This is indeed why holistic dentists believe emphatically in prevention starting before birth and continuing meticulously through the years. Children who experience dental traumas, and I consider anything more than just a quick look and probe at the teeth a trauma, are likely to react badly to the dentist and may develop phobias relating to the care of their teeth in the future. There is inevitable child variation, of course, with some children perfectly happy to accept treatment that is dependent on good parental attitudes and a good, considerate dentist, but on average no one, neither child nor adult, finds any sort of dental treatment pleasant, and therefore prevention should be of paramount importance from the beginning.

The use of fluoride drops and fluoride tablets is considered a major aspect of prevention at this deciduous stage. Fluoride is undoubtedly effective against tooth decay, but holistic practitioners feel that it is difficult to measure the amount of fluoride being ingested. With fluoride in some water supplies, in toothpastes, and occurring naturally in some foods, ingestion may be too great, and staining of teeth, etc., can occur. Potentially more seriously, though, is the effect the fluoride might have on the growing bones and tissues of the body.

Ingested fluoride has an effect on all calcifying tissue, especially growing bones, as well as forming teeth. If fluoride is ingested in large amounts, what effect is it having on the growing bones of a child? The answer is that no one really knows, and this is the holistic argument against fluoride. If the effect on the body of any substance is not precisely or accurately known, then the body should not ingest it artificially.

From a balanced reading of arguments both for and against fluoride,[72] I am an agnostic. I know the undoubted dental benefits of fluoride but, not knowing the long-term effects of drops or tablets taken in these first few growing years, I could not possibly advocate their use. This is not because I believe it is harmful; it is because I just do not know. If in doubt, don't!

Topical fluoride can be useful, though, at this stage. It is painted directly onto the tooth enamel, where it can do good without having any effect on the rest of the body. However, it is not safe to use on too young of a child, as he will not be able to prevent himself from swallowing the toothpaste.

Again, to take a holistic approach, if the diet is adequate, then the teeth should be safe from decay without the additional help of fluoride. The use of fluoride assumes that the teeth will decay; therefore, aiming to make them harder and more resistant is treating the effect, not the cause. With good diet and a sound nutritional

---

72 (a) http://blogs.mercola.com/sites/vitalvotes/archive/2007/06/11/Finally--Even-Dental-Association-Agrees-Fluoride-is-Bad.aspx
(b) http://www.guardian.co.uk/science/2008/feb/09/medicalresearch.health—"Fluoride, Teeth, and an Argument That's Full of Holes," by Ben Goldacre, MD
(c) http://www.nofluoride.com/Unicef_fluor.htm - UNICEF's Position on Water Fluoridation

Great Teeth for Life

base starting before the baby is born, we could claim that a child should not develop tooth decay.

Thumb Sucking and Other Habits

Sucking is such a basic instinct for a baby that it can start in the womb. Scans have shown the near-term baby sucking a thumb or finger. It is associated in the earliest days with the pleasure of feeding, and thereafter it can be a comfort at times of stress, hunger, or tiredness. Up to the age of about seven, the comfort value often outweighs the potential damage to the jaws, but equally it should never be actively encouraged.

From about seven years and older, thumb sucking should be actively discouraged. The pressure of the thumb and the sucking action can lead to a class 2 appearance, i.e., the upper jaw is protrusive and the lower jaw pushed back. This often requires extensive orthodontic work and can also lead to jaw problems. The dentist can advise on ways in which a child can be weaned off thumb sucking, and an orthodontic appliance is often the best form of habit breaker.

When children suck their thumb or fingers, this can occasionally cause the teeth to take on abnormal shapes where they have been depressed or worn away by the constant repetitive action. The deciduous teeth can wear away right up to the gum line, often showing a sort of halo effect, for baby teeth are not as durable as the permanent teeth. Once the enamel has been breached, the underlying dentin is relatively soft and can erode away quickly.

In this situation, dental advice would normally be that there is nothing to worry about. The teeth are not permanent, and this will not affect the permanent teeth waiting to erupt, as long as care is taken and potentially damaging habits are stopped in time.

Accidental Damage to a Baby Tooth

When babies start to walk, they are unsteady and can easily fall down. Subsequently, up to the period of mixed dentition, at about the age of six, they are exploring their world and have little fear, and this is when many accidents can happen. Luckily, nature has compensated for this in a number of ways.

The jawbone is more flexible, allowing bumps and bangs to be cushioned more than in a mature jaw. The baby teeth are protected in such a way that they can sustain a much greater degree of damage than the permanent teeth can. A baby tooth can be quite severely displaced during a fall, but within a couple of days, it often grows back into its previous position, guided by the action of the tongue and cheeks.

Generally, the pulps of baby teeth are well supplied with blood vessels, nerves, etc., and the apical foramen are often quite large. This is where the tooth joins the bone—and where all the nerves and blood vessels flow from the bone into the tooth. When a baby tooth is damaged, there is often a bruising—the tooth will actually look gray or black—but within a couple of weeks, this coloration gradually disappears and the tooth tightens up and becomes white again. This is because of the good supply of blood inside the tooth, which can wash away the bruised tissue and allow new healthy nerve endings and the blood supply to be replaced inside the tooth. This doesn't always happen, of course, and the tooth can die if the damage is too great.

Care during the Mixed Dentition Period

In baby dentition, the full arc of twenty teeth will normally be complete by two and a half years. We then have a period of rest dentally until about the age of six, when there are often the first signs of eruption of the first permanent molars. With the arrival of these teeth, we enter the era of what is called mixed dentition, when the jaw contains both baby teeth and permanent teeth in the mouth at the same time.

From Baby Teeth to Permanent Teeth

This is the beginning of a time of continual change, which goes on for years: from six to eight, a lot is happening; from eight to ten, there's typically a lull. Then, from ten to twelve, there is a great deal of activity again. This is "teething" in the real sense, filling the mouth with teeth that will be utilized for a lifetime, and it can cause discomfort in the early stages, although it's ironic that no one ever attributes a six-year-old's moods to teething!

From the ages of six to twelve, a small mouth can often look like a hodgepodge, with gaps, half-grown teeth, and what sometimes looks like double or treble rows of teeth. If the jaw is wide enough and grows well, then everything should sort itself out normally throughout this period. In the Western world, however, due to both diet and genetics, there are problems, and orthodontic treatment is often necessary.

The body during this time is undertaking periods of growth, usually in spurts, and it is the same with the teeth. As with the eruption of deciduous teeth, the timing for the loss of baby teeth and the eruption of permanent teeth is all a matter of genetic variation, and there are no definitive rules.

The first to appear are usually the molars at the back, between six and eight years of age, and subsequently there is a loss of the lower incisors, followed by the lower laterals. Next are the upper central and lateral incisors. When this has been attained, by about eight and a half years, there is a period of rest and no further loss of teeth until the child is about ten years old. This is when the lower baby canines fall out and are replaced by the permanent canines.

The other permanent teeth all erupt during the next few years, until about age thirteen, excluding the third molars that generally erupt from about seventeen to twenty-one years of age. The timings are not always related to these ages because growth hormones can possibly play a part as well. The growth spurts generally associated with boys and girls at the onset of puberty could coincide with spurts in tooth growth as well, and it's not uncommon for children of fourteen or fifteen years old to still have some baby teeth, which, on average, should have been gone at about twelve years of age (see charts on page 71).

The first permanent teeth to erupt are usually the first molars. These do not take the place of any of the other baby teeth, but erupt farther behind or at the back of the last baby molars, the Es (see chart on page 71). This eruption can be accompanied by some discomfort, as these teeth are large, the largest of our molars, and the gum flap that covers them can be quite tough for the tooth to break through. Sometimes there can be what is called an eruption cyst, and this is where the tissue above the tooth fills with fluid and forms a little lump in the mouth. This can look quite alarming, often like a blue-black ball, but it is comparatively painless, and the child can usually burst it by simply biting into it with the opposing teeth. If parents get alarmed, the dentist can quickly lance it, and the tooth will then erupt quite normally on its own.

As the permanent tooth grows underneath the baby tooth, the osteoclasts will "eat" the baby root, the permanent tooth will move farther up into the inverted U-shape, and the baby tooth, loosened by its diminishing root structure, will start to wobble and eventually come out. Children can then work the loose tooth with their tongues (many adults still talk about the pleasures of inserting a tongue into the side of a loose baby tooth to encourage it on its way), and this "helping hand" is not a bad thing. A loose tooth present for too long can mean bacteria and trapped food debris. It should not be encouraged when a tooth has hardly any mobility. As many children can be overenthusiastic about baby teeth loss, thinking about the money left under the pillow by the tooth fairy, this is a useful way of making the loss and changeover of teeth into a happy and interesting event for both parent and child.

[NB: Inflation has meant that when I started practice, the tooth fairy left 2.5 pence; now it is at least one pound!]

Sometimes, though, when permanent teeth erupt to the side of baby teeth, giving the appearance of a double row or "banking" of teeth, the baby teeth can take a little longer to fall out. In extreme cases, when they are very stubborn and preventing the permanent tooth from moving into its correct position, a dentist may need to give that final push, perhaps by extraction (the one time when the removal of a baby tooth by "unnatural" means could be beneficial).

Great Teeth for Life

The permanent tooth will then move into its designated place by the action of tongue and cheeks. Sometimes a permanent tooth can erupt earlier than expected, when a baby tooth is missing because of accident or extraction, and the permanent tooth doesn't have the opposition of dissolving away the root of the baby tooth.

Throughout this period, when the activity is so high, cleaning the teeth properly is difficult, and parents must scrupulously oversee it. There are irregularities not just in the position of the teeth, but also in the height of the teeth, with some baby teeth being pushed and tilted by the permanent teeth underneath. With the additional hazards of loose teeth and some inevitable crowding, it is a time when children are most vulnerable to tooth decay and dental infections.

It is also a time when sweet eating might be at its height, even if parents have scrupulously avoided sweet things at home; especially when children start school, they'll inevitably encounter them. The avoidance of sugars and rigorous cleaning needs to be strictly maintained, as well as the use of topical fluoride, which will be soaked up by the more porous enamel of the new teeth and give protection.

Altogether, the whole process of transition from baby teeth to permanent teeth is a remarkable one. It is usually very rapid in biological terms, and it all goes astonishingly smoothly considering all the things that can go wrong. At this time, the mouth and jaw are in constant turmoil, in a constant state of activity, and most children seem to cope with teething, and there is a normal and predictable pattern. However, things can and do go wrong, and this is probably when the orthodontist steps in.

Planning Orthodontics

Orthodontics and mixed dentition go together and are inextricably linked. Through orthodontic awareness at an early age, a dentist can plan in advance and obviate many potentially distressing problems. A dentist, hand in glove with a caring parent, will have seen the development of his youthful patient; will be monitoring general growth in tandem with growth of jaws; and will be overseeing the transition from deciduous to permanent teeth. A conscientious dentist, not necessarily holistic, should start planning orthodontically as soon as any potential problem first reveals itself.

The study and practice of orthodontics, which is the regulation or straightening of teeth, has become an important part of progressive and preventative dentistry. Although I believe that diet plays a major role in ensuring that jaw and teeth form to their maximum growth potential, orthodontics is becoming increasingly relevant in an imperfect world. By having good straight teeth through orthodontic planning and treatment, the patient will be happier with his appearance and will, hopefully, pay more attention to the care of his teeth in the future.

If teeth are straight and not too tightly crammed together, they will be easier to clean. If toothbrush filaments and floss can easily reach in between the teeth, bacteria will not gather, and the likelihood of disease will be diminished

Orthodontic treatment can entail the use of appliances such as braces and may require the extraction of teeth. It all depends on the individual mouth of the child. By keeping a close watch on developments, a dentist, who will either initiate the orthodontic plan or do so in tandem with a specialist orthodontist, can fairly accurately predict what will happen in terms of jaw expansion and the size of teeth, together with potential crowding. In order to obtain the full orthodontic picture, X-rays may need to be taken. Although holistically I am reluctant to consider radiation in relation to growing tissue and bones, this is a time when it may be vital. The dentist will be able to examine the size, position, and angle of the jaws, as well as the situation of the permanent teeth, to see if there are too many or too few, and plan accordingly. A relatively recent development in orthodontic treatment is the potential for expanding the jaw, as opposed to diminishing it by extraction.

Most orthodontic treatment does not start until the child is about eleven or twelve years old. It can be started earlier, but this may involve the removal of baby teeth, which I am not in favor of unless absolutely necessary. It can also involve what we call "serial extractions," when perhaps several baby teeth are removed at the sides to make the front four teeth look better. This may help temporarily, but it doesn't alleviate the orthodontic problem, and it will mean more extraction when the permanent teeth grow.

Serial extractions were popular some years ago, but many consultant orthodontists now have different views, thinking more about the psychology of the child than of the ideal textbook orthodontic situation. A child who has perhaps been very dentally fit, and who is faced with extractions at seven to eight, followed by more at eleven or twelve, will not have positive ideas about treatment at the dentist, and may become reluctant to wear braces.

Parents should never be frightened to seek advice from their dentists, especially when the child is in the eight- to ten-year-old age group. Planning, followed by treatment at about eleven or twelve, is preferable. If orthodontic treatment is left until the child is, for example, fourteen, she may be reluctant to have her appearance marred by braces, and she could indeed be subject to ridicule from her friends. Recently, however, fixed orthodontic appliances have gathered a fashion status, with children asking for fixed appliances—long may this trend continue! Getting the teeth right at this stage will ensure a good dentition for the rest of the child's life, with a good appearance and less disease. Holistically speaking, anyone who is proud of the appearance of his or her teeth will cherish and look after them.

Color of Teeth

Teeth come in shades of all colors, almost literally, but pure white is rare, believe it or not. Dentists who have to make crowns are required to match colors of teeth, and they use shade guides relying on, in dental terms, many separate color variations. The most common shades are of gray, yellow, brown, or, yes, orange! Using these four colors as a basis, with variations and tints on each, most people will fit into these categories.

The actual color of a tooth depends on its thickness. If a front tooth is thin, the tooth will have a more translucent appearance and will often appear grayer. Indeed, if you look closely, as a dentist has to in order to match shades for crowns, the various shades of blue or pink can show through due to the translucency of the tooth!

It is at the mixed dentition stage that parents begin to feel worried about the color of their children's teeth. For example, when a child has two new permanent front teeth, they can look discolored in comparison to the baby teeth. These do often look whiter because they're smaller, and also due to the amount of calcium from which they're composed. Parents can normally be reassured that once all the permanent teeth are through, the color will look uniform and of good quality.

Other color worries could indeed be justified due to a tetracycline prescribed during pregnancy or infancy, or to fluorosis. A tooth that is grayer in color than others, whether deciduous or permanent, could be due to tooth death after a knock. New permanent front teeth often have areas of hypocalcification where little spots, blotches, or stripes of color, usually white, are clearly visible. These may become less conspicuous as the other teeth grow, in that they will all look uniform, but the imperfections may be permanent, due perhaps to abnormalities of nutrition of the tooth at a crucial early stage.

Replanting Teeth

Just as the two- to six-year-old stage is fairly adventurous, so are the later stages, when children seem never to have any fear or take any care. This is a time when a permanent tooth may be knocked out, and this is much more serious. If the child can be rushed to the dentist with the tooth kept moist (best in milk, not necessarily organic, as water can have an adverse osmotic effect on the tooth and milk seems to be gentler), then often the tooth can be replanted by the dentist. Sometimes the tooth will reattach to the jawbone but the pulp inside the tooth will die.

With the advances of current science, however, when severed arms have been sewn back on successfully, the future possibilities of cell growth and stimulation cannot be entirely dismissed. Currently, dentists are relying on a process similar to root filling, and this sort of transplantation can work reasonably well for up to ten years.[73]

73 (a) Andersson, L.; Bodin I. "Avulsed Human Teeth Replanted Within 15 Minutes—A long-term clinical follow-up study." *Dental Traumatology*,

Great Teeth for Life

A permanent tooth that is knocked out is a shame, but it need not be a permanent disaster, and it can occasionally be the basis of a new, improved, and less destructive orthodontic plan. Why take out more sound teeth when an accident has already deprived the mouth of one! So, following such trauma, the dentist also makes an orthodontic assessment.

Permanent Teeth

Although many adults nowadays may have crooked or crowded teeth, our children can now have perfect jaws, teeth, and dental arches because of good nutrition, better hygiene, caring dentistry, and efficient orthodontic treatment. That the latter may depend on a couple of years of minor discomfort, and a less than exciting appearance if braces are worn, should never be allowed to matter. The future of the teeth that are needed for the rest of life is at stake.

Parents can still play a supportive and encouraging role at this stage, and indeed the teenage years, when children may perhaps rebel to a certain extent over a number of issues, including nutrients, which can be very destructive to the teeth. This is a time when diet can be poor indeed, with fizzy drinks, fast foods, cookies, sugary snacks, and cakes to assuage the hungers that assail teenagers. As a result, tooth decay can set in on the permanent teeth during these years. Most people who require dental fillings in their twenties and thirties will have laid the foundations of that decay when in their teens.

Although it may be difficult for parents to make their voices heard, they should still try to help in a number of ways. A continuing good diet at home will help offset the new dietary temptations that present themselves when teenagers have money of their own. An earlier taught dental hygiene regime will hopefully carry on as habit. Encouragement to visit the dentist regularly will be another major factor in prevention.

---

27 April 2006, Dept of Oral Surgery, Carolinska Hospital, Stockholm, Sweden. http://www3.interscience.wiley.com/journal/118537215/home (b) Floria, G. "Orthodontic Splints in Dental Traumatology." Firenze, Italy, http://www.vjo.it/two/splint.htm

Brian Halvorsen, BDS, LDS RCS

Wisdom Teeth

These are the last of our permanent teeth, and they can influence the dentition from about the age of sixteen, although they may not erupt until the later teens or early twenties. In fact, I knew someone who was seventy before his erupted! Historically, wisdom teeth were the "reserves." When primitive man wore down his teeth by chewing and grinding on abrasive foods, the teeth became smaller in height and width, and moved toward the front of the mouth. Dentists call this movement mesial drift, which is thought to be nature's way of allowing room for the reserves to grow into the mouth. Nowadays, we lack abrasive foods, and our teeth don't wear down, yet there's still the mesial drift to allow for the wisdom teeth. Both the mesial drift and the teeth themselves can cause problems.

The mesial drift occurs even without wisdom teeth, and this can affect orthodontic treatment. If, at the age of fifteen, the teeth have been orthodontically persuaded into a lovely, even arch, then the mesial drift can undo all that work, making the teeth tighten together again, even sometimes overlapping. The dentist should always monitor the potential of this carefully because it would be a shame to have a wonderfully aesthetic result at the age of fifteen, which developed into a crowded mess at twenty.

The wisdom teeth are almost superfluous to our needs nowadays, and jaws have become smaller anyway. Often the answer is extraction, both from the orthodontic point of view and because they can undoubtedly cause problems. They can erupt in a bad position, jammed against the tooth in front, or into the bone, or into the tissue and muscle at the end of the gum ridge simply because there isn't room for them.

This pressure can cause pain in itself, but there could also be a space between the wisdom tooth and the swollen gum in which food and bacteria could collect, which can often cause inflammation, infection, and pain. Any wisdom teeth will probably have to be removed as a result. Indeed, calling them "wisdom teeth" is a misnomer, as for most of us, it is anything but wise to have them!

CHAPTER FIVE

Tooth Decay—Sweet Tooth/Rotten Tooth!

At the very least, tooth decay can be painful, disfiguring, and extremely expensive. In Britain, dentists perform at least thirty million fillings annually. If this seems outrageous, you should note that this figure only includes treatments in England and Wales. Scotland lists its figures separately, and both sets of figures are those recorded by the National Health Service and do not including private patients, which will add a considerable number. These figures must also be seen in relation to the number of people who go to the dentist on a regular basis, which is well known to be no more than 50 percent of the population. Considering all these figures, it means that there was at least one filling for every person who went to the dentist! These fillings are, and were, the result of tooth decay.

The cost to the dental part of the National Health Service in 2008 to 2009 was in excess of two billion pounds ($3.24 billion),[74] and much of that would have been expended on tooth decay. This figure is only what it cost us as a nation; it does not include the cost of productive time lost by people attending the dentist.

To take the concept even further, the enormous financial cost does not include the valuable learning hours lost by schoolchildren, the equally valuable work and leisure hours lost by adults and children alike, nor indeed the hours that dentists could be utilizing much more effectively with dietary and hygiene instruction, i.e., prevention.

Did I forget to mention the dreadful hours of pain and disaster tooth decay can inflict? All this money, time, and discomfort is being

---

74 "BDA (British Dental Association) Gives 'Qualified Welcome' to NHS Dentistry Budget Increase," UK, Dec 2007, Pater Ward, Chief Executive of the BDA http://www.medicalnewstoday.com/arti cles/92433.php

expended on a disease that is largely preventable. It is undeniable that with a combination of good diet, good hygiene techniques, and fluoride therapy, tooth decay could be virtually eliminated.

In fact, since treatments were recorded, it can truthfully be said that the levels of tooth decay in Britain have fallen. Besides the efforts of dentists and their teams, this decrease is also due to the work of the local dental authorities and, surprisingly, toothpaste and toothbrush manufacturers.

Not only have they included fluoride in their toothpastes, but they have also distributed informative and invaluable literature and preventative programs to dentists, schools, and clinics, and the dental profession should be grateful to them for this. The public is now much better informed as a result, and has become so at a much earlier age, which is vital in terms of effective prevention.

The Role of Sugar in Tooth Decay

As saliva plus bacteria equals plaque, so it can be said that plaque plus sugar equals acid, which in turn causes tooth decay. As with anything, it is never quite that simple. Every one of us can probably point to an individual who eats sweets all day, never brushes his or her teeth, never goes to the dentist, and who never seems to develop any tooth decay. Equally, we all know of people who are dentally very conscientious, and yet who suffer endlessly from decay problems. Sadly, it is a fact that some people are just more vulnerable to decay than others are. This could be hereditary or genetic, but it is primarily a matter of individual biochemistry. It could be that the enamel did not calcify properly; it could be that the major acid-producing bacteria are much more prolific in a particular mouth; or it could be a combination of factors. Fermentable carbohydrates (sugars) will always be implicated.

The breakdown of the biochemistry in an individual mouth can be likened to those dominos, which are made to fall down in progression. Even if only one of the mouth factors already mentioned alters, or is altered, in some way—e.g., the oral bacteria, the shape of the teeth, the content and flow of the saliva, the way in which the mouth is used—then the delicate interaction is altered. The dominos start to fall, and tooth decay could be the result.

But sugar, of course, despite individual variances in vulnerability and resistance, is still the principal cause of tooth decay. The interaction with plaque in the mouth starts the whole process. The theory of caries, or tooth decay, is attributed to one W. B. Millar. At the end of the last century, he incubated teeth with saliva and carbohydrates. Acid formed, and the enamel of the teeth dissolved. When carbohydrate was excluded, no dissolution took place, and so he concluded that carbohydrate was needed to cause tooth decay.

The Sugar That We Eat

Sugar is a carbohydrate, along with the starches, and starch carbohydrates are valuable to the body in that they are a useful and often cheap source of energy. The unrefined complex carbohydrates found in vegetables, fruit, pulses, and whole grains are the best type that you can eat because they are combined with vitamins, minerals, and trace elements, as well as dietary fiber. Most carbohydrates in a Western diet, however, have been so refined and concentrated that they are virtually empty foods, stripped of any nutritional value.

The most empty carbohydrate of all is processed white sugar, for it provides only calories and nothing else whatsoever, and it is actually added to a vast number of "foods." Sugar could truthfully be described as one of the major evils of civilization, for it is hazardous to our health in so many ways, as well as its undoubted dental effect. Sugar has been directly linked with a multitude of other medical problems. In fact, as one well-known expert has said, if sugar were to be marketed as a drug, it would be banned immediately!

All the sugars that we eat are potentially harmful from a dental point of view, but the most dangerous are the most refined, the stickiest and the powdered. Even the natural sugars found in fruit and vegetables (fructose) and milk (lactose) could, if conditions in the mouth were bad enough, lead to acid production, for virtually any carbohydrate, even the non-sugar starches, can eventually, if given long enough, produce acid that then produces tooth decay.

Other sugars that are considered more natural are honey and the unrefined cane sugars. They do undoubtedly contain many good things nutritionally, such as minerals and vitamins, etc.[75] However, dentally they are just as damaging, particularly honey, as it can remain on the teeth for longer.

The more refined a sugar, the less nutritious and the more detrimental it becomes. The gleaming white crystal table sugar that is sprinkled on cereals or stirred into hot drinks, and the icing sugar that makes cake frostings, are the worst of all. If you consider that the average amount of sugar eaten per week by every man, woman, and child in the United Kingdom is at least two pounds (900 grams), then it comes as no surprise that we are still ravaged by the horrors of tooth decay. In the United States, sugar consumption has increased to an average of 135 pounds (62 kilograms) per person per annum[76].

Although the consumption of white sugar has dropped, the consumption of confectionery has increased. Sugar may have been dropped from tea or coffee, but a sweet craving for sugar is addictive, and it still continues and is being satisfied by confectionery. About four ounces (110 grams) of those two pounds of sugar is consumed in the form of confectionery. Children consume twice the national average of sweets and therefore can consume up to eight ounces (225 grams) of sugar per week. Some children eat up to eight ounces of sugar every day! As children are especially vulnerable to tooth decay, what with mass advertising and the availability of sweet things, they can also become victims of obesity and early diabetes. During World War II, when sugar was either rationed

---

75 (a) "Healthful Honey," Chemistry of Honey, 2005 Michigan, USA www.honey-health.com/honey-5.shtml
   (b) Tozian, G. "On the Sweet Tooth of a Dilemma," Organicanews.com, 1997 http://www.organicanews.com/news/article.cfm?story_id=23
   (c) http://www.mcvitamins.com/Health%20Opponents/cane-juice.htm - as (b)

76 "Sugar's Effect on Your Health," *Healing Daily*, 2007, http://www.healingdaily.com/detoxification-diet/sugar.htm

or not available, the incidence of new cases of diabetes dropped substantially, but then it increased when sugar was freely available after the war.[77]

It is social conditioning to believe that sweets are a "treat." A more truthful statement would be that sweets are a "poison," and any product that contains a large percentage of sugar, 10 percent, for example, should carry the message DANGER: HEALTH WARNING. THIS PRODUCT CONTAINS SUGAR, WHICH CAN SERIOUSLY DAMAGE YOUR HEALTH, just as on cigarette packets. We could also tax sweets, for they are basically a nonnutritious food, and profits could go toward anti-sugar advertising. Perhaps the day might come when sugar and sweets manufacturers could be sued for the amount of pain and suffering their wares cause.

Not only sweets contain refined sugar. A staggering number of other products contain hidden sugars. Cakes, sweetened cereals, cookies, jams, fruits canned in syrup, even dried fruit, and chocolate drinks are obvious, but less obvious are "health" cereals; bread; canned tomato soup, which contains 10 percent sucrose; ketchup; canned peas, beans, and spaghetti; and corned beef!

You should get into the habit of reading the contents of labels for refined foods—packets, bags, cans, etc.—and the number of unlikely things that contain sugar will amaze you. Remember that, like baby foods, the ingredients are listed in descending order of quantity. Sugar near the top of the list means a large proportion of sugar.

Happily, food labeling is becoming more detailed, but it should list the type of sugar as well, and the percentage of sugar that is present. We could then easily avoid them. Although many supermarket chains are becoming more aware of the public dislike for sugar and other additives, the only way to truly convince all manufacturers is

---

77 (a) Trowell, White Lies, 1974 http://www.vegetarian.org.uk/campaigns/whitelies/wlreport11.shtml
(b) Lieberman, L. "Diabetes Mellitus and Medical Anthropology." Encyclopedia of Medical Anthropology: Topics v. 1: Health and Illness in the World's Cultures, 21 Nov 2006, Ember, C. and Ember, M., eds. New York: Springer, 2003

simply not to buy their goods until they are forced to take sugar out of their products. Remember to read the labels before buying!

There is sugar in many medicines as well, in antibiotics, laxatives, cough syrups, vitamins, and tranquillizers and antidepressants, and it is particularly horrifying that liquid baby medicines are high in sucrose. Manufacturers like to use sugar syrup as a base because it is cheap and masks the principal active ingredients; it also helps the medicine have a longer shelf life. There is obviously an assumption too that babies will more readily take a medicine with a sweet taste, and doctors and dentists should be fighting vigorously against this. There are now some baby medicines that are sugar-free, but of the antibiotics, probably the most commonly prescribed medicine in infancy and childhood, there are, from one survey, twenty-one with sugar and only one without. The good news is that things are improving!

When Sugar Is Most Damaging

A high-sugar diet is one in which sugar is taken at frequent intervals, even if it is in small amounts. The frequency of sugar consumption is what is most damaging in both body and dental terms. One cream cake a week for a treat (although I dislike that word and concept), or in an unavoidable social circumstance, probably won't do a great deal of harm. But the snack foods eaten between meals, when saliva production is low, and the sugar taken in those frequent cups of tea or coffee throughout the day are likely to produce the most acid, and thus the potential for the most teeth decay.

Every time sugar comes in touch with plaque, the acid produced will stay on the teeth for up to twenty minutes. The sugar will not clear from the teeth for that time, and the chart below shows the acidogenicity of some common foods. It's like stoking a boiler. The more sugar that is put in, the more acid will be produced, and the production of acid will go on for longer.

Acidogenicity of Common Snack Foods

Most acidogenic:

Boiled sweets (fruit-flavored)
Sugared coffees
Toffee
Orange drink (sweetened)
Plain biscuit (sweet)
Sugared chewing gum
Chocolate biscuit
Sweet chocolate
Ice cream
Cream-filled biscuit
Apple
Chocolate/caramel bar
Chocolate covered peanuts
Cough syrup
Unsweetened coffee
Ice lolly (frozen fruit drink)
Potato crisps/chips
Bread and butter
Peanuts

Least acidogenic:

Sugar-free chewing gum

Adapted from the work of W. M. Edgar, reproduced in *Diet, Nutrition and Dentistry* **by Randolph and Dennison (The C. V. Mosby Company, 1981)**
[NB: Although this list is from nearly thirty years ago, nothing has really changed!]

Smokers who suck mint sweets regularly to freshen their breath (and sucking is worse than chewing) are prone to this prolonged acid attack, and when they give up smoking, it can be even worse in their new need for an alternative oral stimulation! If a mint is sucked every ten minutes throughout the day, the effects in terms of acid production will be worse than if ten packets of mints were consumed all in one go. Similarly, it is no good for people to claim that they only have one teaspoon of sugar in each drink if they actually have ten cups of coffee per day. They would be better off having one cup containing ten teaspoons of sugar!

The consistency of sugar is also a consideration, and the dentist's horror is the chocolate-coated soft caramel bar that is sticky and full of sucrose. The consistency of the sucrose will lower the pH of the mouth much more drastically because it dissolves so quickly (which is why fizzy drinks are so bad: the sucrose is already dissolved). The stickiness of the sucrose will contribute similarly to a rapid lowering of the pH and will also stick to the plaque on the tooth for longer. The saliva will not be able to wash it away so easily.

Although sugar is undeniably bad for teeth and for health in general, there is another aspect of sugar consumption that is extremely worrying. All carbohydrates can supply energy, and most of them do so more nutritiously than white sugar. Many sugar-eating children are gaining their energy solely from sugarcoated cereals, sweets, and ice creams, and thus are not eating the more nutritious foods.

A classic example is of the child who does not have room for proper meals but who satisfies his hunger and energy needs through eating sugary snack foods. Many children who constantly eat sweet and refined food can be technically as severely malnourished as children who have little or no food at all.

Sugar and Children's Teeth

Tooth decay on baby teeth can be an unmitigated disaster. This must be one of the worst ways in which sugar can work its dreadful effects, and thus sugar should be avoided at all costs. Decay can be caused by pacifiers dipped in honey, which are constantly in the mouth. Other villains are the sweet syrupy drinks for children, perhaps left in a feeding bottle for the baby or child to suck.

A small amount of tooth decay on a baby tooth can cause considerable damage. The teeth are small so that a tiniest cavity can damage the nerve or cause an abscess. Once the cavity is established, the tooth can quickly degenerate and break down because the structure of the deciduous enamel is thinner and the dentin weaker than a permanent tooth.

Teeth that decay at an early age might need filling more than once by the time they are eventually lost, and the psychological effects of these treatments on a young four- or five-year-old child can be distressing. Avoidance of sugar during the period of deciduous dentition is vital, as the teeth are not designed to go bad.

Tooth decay can seriously affect the first permanent molars, usually the first teeth to erupt at about the age of six. The tooth is more porous and much more chemically active at this age. Good and bad chemicals can affect the surface enamel. Sugar at this rather vital stage, the time when children start to demand sweets (perhaps coinciding with going to school), can be disastrous, as holes may appear virtually overnight—i.e., the first permanent molars can decay rapidly; these teeth should be a lifetime's investment. This is when topical fluoride could be applied, as it will more effectively soak into the new tooth's surface. It's rather like painting a rough unseasoned piece of wood, when the first coat literally soaks into the untreated surface. A dental history of decay in the baby teeth should warn the dentist that these permanent teeth are also at risk as they erupt.

The avoiding of sugar is still the greatest priority. Sugar control is more important in preventing tooth decay than any other measure. As a profession, we have been lobbying for years, but against the bureaucratic and financial might of the opposing lobby, the sugar and sweet manufacturers, to whom the United Kingdom consumption of sugar is 2.25 million tons per year, our voices echo in the wilderness. As a result, our main effort has been diverted into looking at ways of preventing tooth decay, and thus the use of fluoride.

It is a fudging of the issue and treating of the effects, not the cause. The principal thrust of prevention still ought to be the elimination of refined sugar entirely from everyone's diet. However, a sensible goal at this stage would be to aim for a realistic reduction in both the quantity and frequency of the refined sugar intake.

The Progression of Tooth Decay

Water on the untreated metal of a car produces a chemical reaction that dissolves the surface of the metal. The rust may only reveal itself at first as a few small bubbles on the surface, but once the paint is stripped away, there could be a massive amount of rust and destruction beneath. Similarly, decay on a tooth, which may look minimal, could have spread underneath the enamel, throughout the dentin, to create a much more destructive cavity.

The Early Stages and Remineralisation

Early tooth decay is in essence a demineralization of the tooth's surface. The acid dissolves the minerals from the enamel. The plaque has the capacity to soak up vast amounts of calcium and can draw minerals from the tooth surface. At this early stage; visible signs might be little white spots on the enamel; the effects at this stage may not be felt at all; or the tooth might react to hot or cold, especially the latter.

This is the time when there is a two-way process involving the ebb and flow of minerals, which can affect tooth decay and its progression. Once this early tooth decay is present, it does not mean that it necessarily has to get worse. If the body and mouth environment changes or is adjusted correctly, primarily through a good diet, within days the saliva can deposit more minerals to replace those taken out. Through a good diet and the use of topical fluoride, these spots of early tooth decay can be slowed or stopped. There is a good chance that the tooth can regenerate and repair itself. This is called "remineralization."

Cavities

Once the acid breaches the enamel and reaches the dentin, however, cavities are created, bacteria can wreak their toxic havoc, and dental fillings will probably be necessary. That's when the dentist has to make up his mind what the next step might be. If there is a tiny cavity, it may remain static. If a good diet and meticulous hygiene were followed, the early cavity could be observed and merely checked at every visit to see if it has grown any larger. This is a decision the dentist has to make, weighing up the general body and mouth condition of the patient in order to assess the rate of tooth decay.

Once a cavity is big enough for the bacteria to live in, it can begin to have a toxic effect, and it is no longer just the acid produced that is damaging. Bacteria are in a sheltered haven, out of reach of the toothbrush, floss, and toothpaste, where there is plenty of fermentable carbohydrate constantly reaching into the cavity. At this stage, the bacteria can feed at leisure and without fear of being removed, and although the saliva can reach in, it has to do so through a jungle of bacteria and food debris. The more the "cave" effect of the cavity, the more the bacteria has free rein and the greater the likelihood that a filling will be required.

The most likely parts of the tooth to decay are the areas that are difficult to clean thoroughly: the fissures on the biting surfaces of the molars, in between tight teeth or merely teeth that touch each other, and the border between teeth and gums. Tooth decay can occur on the top of teeth, at the sides, or between—in fact, anywhere that plaque is allowed to accumulate. If undetected and left to multiply, the bacteria will spread rapidly through the dentin and pass along its tiny canals to infect the pulp at the heart of the tooth.

Abscesses

Fig. 12
Tooth Decay and Abscess

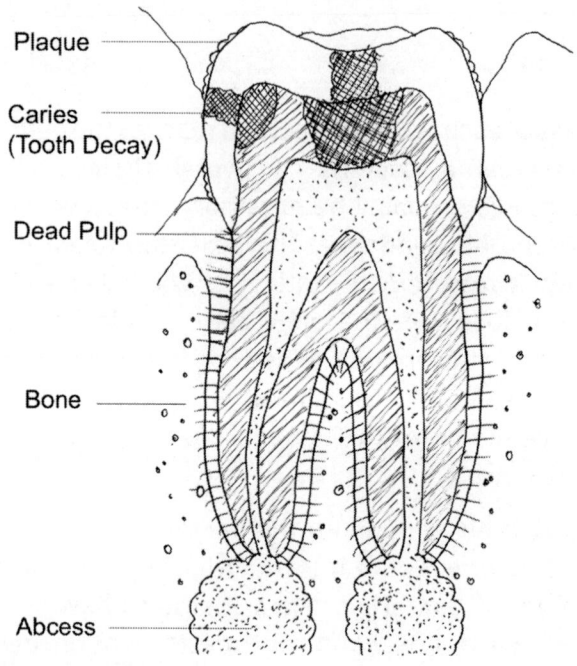

Labels: Plaque, Caries (Tooth Decay), Dead Pulp, Bone, Abcess

Illustrated by Caroline White
Copyright held by Brian Halvorsen
Credit:
Illustrations by Caroline White, copyright Brian Halvorsen 2010.

A tooth abscess occurs when the bacteria and the putrefying products and toxins of decay kill the nerve of the tooth; in the vast majority of cases, this is due to tooth decay, or the consequences of having a tooth damaged or filled, and the tooth may not die at the time. Dead and dying nerve tissue expands, leaving the nerve chamber and infecting the surrounding jawbone. Pus gathers and inflammation spreads, often accompanied by a facial coloring and swelling. Dental abscesses, if allowed to spread, can be very serious. Periodontal abscesses are covered under "Gum Disease."

In the upper jaw, the manner of drainage for infected tissue is often upward, and it can run perilously close to brain tissue. Infection can join vessels that run into the brain, causing infection and possible death. Similarly, in the lower jaw, the swelling in the neck following a dental abscess could be so severe that it obstructs the airway and can cause death through asphyxiation.

This, however, is unlikely in civilized Western society, where dentists and doctors are available to relieve pain and to control infection. A severe dental infection was a cause of death before the advent of antibiotics. Although holistic practitioners do not believe in the use of drugs unless absolutely necessary, antibiotics may be of the essence when attempting to control a dental abscess. In some situations, a dentist can lance an abscess if it's on the surface, allowing the pus to drain out into the mouth. Often, however, the pus will burrow its way inwards through the bone so that the dentist cannot see it or treat it other than by antibiotics. Drilling a hole in the tooth to the nerve chamber can reduce pain by relieving pressure and creating a drain.

Rampant Tooth Decay

Rampant tooth decay occurs when there is little or no remineralization. It is all a one-way process. The teeth are destroyed at a rapid rate. The bacteria inside a tooth multiply phenomenally quickly and physically eat away the interior and surface of the tooth. The nerve can be exposed quickly because it doesn't have time to lay down the protective secondary dentin, and large chunks of the tooth can break off under pressure.

The actual color and texture of rampant tooth decay are different from the more slowly developing ordinary tooth decay. The texture is often soft and cheese-like, and it is also much lighter in color. In ordinary tooth decay, a dentist would have to use a slow drill to remove the decay away in layers. In rampant tooth decay, the dentist can literally scoop the decay out of the tooth. Rampant tooth decay often shows itself as a tiny hole on the surface, and because of its lighter coloration, is often not noticed. Underneath, the tooth is a mess. Rampant tooth decay is both distressing because it is painful, and disfiguring because it can occur in all parts of the mouth, even affecting teeth that are normally much less prone to tooth decay.

Rampant tooth decay is generally related to age and to diet. Individuals who suffer from it often come from deprived backgrounds, which means poor nutrition and bad salivary flow as a result. They can be psychologically disadvantaged as well, with repressed emotions, feelings of inferiority and rebellion, and can be pasty in complexion, and slow learners. This is not a heredity problem, but a nutritional one, where the body and brain just cannot cope with the poor nutrition.

It is also interesting to relate these facts to the recent findings about the relationship between poor diet, mood and personality, and levels of juvenile delinquency.[78] Boys in prison have been shown to change personality when given a good diet after years on a poor one. I expect many of them could have been suffering from rampant tooth decay as well.

However, bad hygiene can also produce rampant tooth decay, as can a diminution of salivary flow. Root caries could almost be called rampant decay, as this occurs in older people who develop a form of diabetes, giving them a constant desire for sweet things. Although their teeth are older and therefore should be more chemically mature and resistant to decay, there is often a lot of root recession, and decay can start there. This root decay progresses quickly, often at a similar rate to rampant tooth decay, and it can result in teeth breaking off, making dental restorations difficult.

Can Tooth Decay Be Contagious?

One person cannot infect another with tooth decay. There are ways in which tooth decay may be regarded as being a transmitted disease. The first is the genetic factor already discussed. It can happen when children inherit a poorer tooth structure or a crowded jaw, and thus a greater vulnerability to tooth decay, from their parents. The second is the

[78] (a) Schoenthaler S., Bier I. "The effect of vitamin-mineral supplementation on juvenile delinquency among American schoolchildren: a randomized, doubleblind placebo-controlled trial." *J Altern Complement Med.* 2000 Feb;6(1):7–17.
(b) Lawrence, J. "Prison Study to Investigate Link Between Junk Food and Violence." *The Independent*, 29th January 2008—http://www.commondreams.org/archive/2008/01/29/6714

acquisition of the wrong bacteria, the image of a hypothetical midwife who might transmit "tooth decay bacteria" to a new baby. Bacteria can be transmitted from mouth to mouth on the breath or by kissing, for example, but it's not a true form of infection, in that most adult mouths will possess the whole range of the same bacteria anyway.

Even if new bacteria were introduced to one mouth, the potential development of tooth decay depends on how that body, mouth, and saliva modify them. Newly acquired bacteria do not necessarily mean a transmitted disease. Even kissing someone who has rampant tooth decay does not mean that the other will develop rampant tooth decay too. But it might be a better idea to point out the unacceptability of rampant tooth decay and refuse to kiss until the sufferer had their teeth seen and treated by a dentist!

The final and major way in which I think one could say that tooth decay is transmittable is through parents feeding their children a bad diet. Parents who allow unlimited access to the tooth decay foods, such as sweets, cookies, cakes, and fizzy drinks are, in effect, infecting their children. They could truly be said to be transmitting disease to their children.

Tooth Decay and Pain

The relationship between tooth decay and pain, surprisingly, is not clear. Dentists often see people with teeth decayed to the gums, teeth reduced to black stumps, teeth with nerves exposed, and teeth with abscesses, but when they ask how severe the discomfort is, the answer often is that the "sufferer" hasn't known a day's pain in his life!

Conversely, a patient can have the smallest early decay mark in a tooth and can feel quite a lot of discomfort. The perception of pain varies enormously from patient to patient, and it must be one of the most difficult and variable sensations to describe and to judge, but it does bear a direct relationship to stress. If someone is under severe stress, it is well known that his pain threshold, the point at which he actually perceives pain, is lowered so that even the smallest stimulus can cause pain. This sounds as if it might be psychological, but it is in fact physical. Biochemical tests have shown that nerve reactions are actually at a higher pitch, and when someone claims that his "nerves are on edge," it is not too far removed from a basic biological truth.

If pain occurs in a tooth, it doesn't necessarily mean the tooth has a hole in it. There are a number of other causes, and even a mild coronary attack could give the sensation of toothache. Too much acidic food and drink, including carbonated water, can give rise to pain and sensitivity.

The symptoms can be the same as early tooth decay, and the solution may be just to use a desensitizing toothpaste, or the dentist can seal over the areas with a desensitizing liquid. Sensitivity can also be caused by overenthusiastic use of the toothbrush or gum recession, but it can also be brought on by stress. If pain were generalized, in more than one part of the mouth, the dentist would be more justified in looking into the cause of the stress, rather than just treating the effects.

The classic decay-related toothache begins when decay extends into the dentin, and bacteria are irritating the nerve tissue. This could cause the early reactions to hot and cold or a minor occasional discomfort. If this is allowed to continue, it will often deteriorate into a pain of longer duration. This is when the decay has spread, and toxins and even bacteria may be entering the nerve of the tooth, and it is followed by a constant pain that can be excruciating. Many have described it as the worst pain that can be perceived. This is often associated with the nerve dying, and once that happens, the severe pain may suddenly cease, to be succeeded by a painless state, or simply a dull sensation. Within a day or two, however, the follow-up could be the characteristic pain of an abscess. This is the time to make an emergency visit to the dentist!

The Prevention of Tooth Decay

Just as even the most minor alteration in one of the chemical factors in the mouth can cause tooth decay, so can the removal of one or more of the factors that contribute to tooth decay make the decay rate decrease dramatically or even cease completely. If hygiene is

Great Teeth for Life

improved, tooth decay can be lessened, and if sugar is omitted from the diet, teeth will be far healthier. By making regular visits to the dentist, incipient tooth decay can be spotted and treated. These basic principles have been reiterated almost ad nauseam, but they are still the major factors in prevention.

Science, too, has been investigating ways of preventing tooth decay. An anti-decay vaccine has been under investigation for at least sixty years, and research has suggested that antibiotics and oral disinfectants can cause a reduction of the bacterial content in the mouth.[79] Many toothpaste manufacturers have been working on enzymes that can inhibit the conversion of carbohydrates into acid. Topical fluoride, too, has an important role in the prevention of tooth decay.

However, from personal experience, from population study research, and from the work of many experts throughout the world,[80] we know that the one overriding factor in low or nonexistent tooth decay appears to be diet. It is the one factor that I feel is relevant and consistent.

Good spacing of teeth, even teeth, and chemically sound teeth are also significant factors in the fight against tooth decay, and they are indirectly the result of good nutrition. The chemistry of the mouth is vital as well, for the saliva is all-important. If the saliva could be rich enough in its preventative factors, it could reduce the bacterial count and inhibit their reproduction. If the saliva has a good flow and viscosity, then there is less tooth decay, due to a more effective detergent effect, with the saliva effectively rinsing the teeth. Saliva is intimately connected with the health of the body in general, and the health of the body is dependent on diet.

The avoidance of sugar is an obvious dietary necessity, and a good whole food diet must be followed. By eating the tough fibrous foods of a good diet—raw fruit and vegetables and whole grains, etc.—

---

79 "The use of Oral Antibiotics and Disinfectants." http://www.jfda.jo
80 (a) Diet and Tooth Decay, 2002, American Dental Association. http://jada.ada.org/cgi/content/full/133/4/527
    (b) World Sugar Research Organization: http://www.wsro.org/public/faqs.html

not only will the health of the body be improved, but the teeth will be cleaned as well. Chewing and chomping can actually have a detergent effect and help the saliva dislodge and wash away much of the bacteria, food debris, and plaque.

The hard bite of people who eat food that is crispy and crunchy can also be a factor. Minerals from the food can be ground into the surface of the tooth, to form a harder, less permeable layer. The pressure and movement can harden up the layers underneath as well, so that the dentin appears thicker and stronger. Heavy mastication can also help prevent tooth decay, as chewing produces more saliva.

The body has an ideal acid/alkaline balance, and the foods that the body ingests, which are either acid or alkaline forming, can affect this balance.

If too many acid-forming foods like coffee, sugar, meat, and processed foods are eaten, they can cause an acid response in the body. This contributes directly to many illnesses such as arthritis; and indeed stress itself produces an acid response in the body. The saliva and oral juices are influenced by the body chemistry, which in turn reduces the saliva's ability to protect the teeth and gums.

If we could produce alkaline reactions in the body through alkaline-forming foods such as fresh raw fruit and vegetables, we might be able to produce alkaline saliva that could combat any acidic effects more effectively.

To summarize, in general, we must always remember that tooth decay is an entirely preventable disease. Provided there is regular attendance at the dentist, a good diet is followed, and oral hygiene is effective (don't forget to consult your dentist or hygienist for an individual program), no one should ever need to have too much dental treatment or lose a tooth through decay.

Despite all this, you might take a horse to water, but you can't make it drink! Unfortunately, there seems to be a resistance to advice, and so we still have dental disease. It is not because there is a lack of information; it is the lack of putting that information into practice. Tooth decay, therefore, is still relevant, and unless there

Great Teeth for Life

is a complete change of heart from everyone, it will remain so into the foreseeable future.

This is not just the situation in England; Australian Prime Minister John Howard has described tooth decay in young children in Australia as a "national tragedy."[81] The disease of tooth decay is truly global, and the United States is following a similar trend![82]

---

81 Australian Associated Press, December 2006, http://www.news.com.au/story/0,27574,20994155-421,00.html

82 (a) Sydney Morning Herald, Australia, Dec 31 2006, "A glass a day to keep decay at bay," http://www.smh.com.au/news/national/a-glass-a-day-to-keep-decay-at-bay-howard/2006/12/30/1166895522686.html
(b) Moles, D.; Ashley, P. Hospital admissions for dental care in children: England 1997–2006. http://www.telegraph.co.uk/health/healthnews/5132883/Rise-in-children-admitted-to-hopistal-with-rotting-death.html
(c) ORAL HEALTH
Preventing Cavities, Gum Disease, and Tooth Loss, At A Glance 2009, Center for Disease Control and Prevention, http://www.cdc.gov/nccdphp/publications/aag/doh.htm

CHAPTER SIX

What's All the Fuss about Fluoride?

It is ironic that the relationship fluoride has with our teeth was not discovered through its beneficial effects but because it can cause unsightly stains and mottling (fluorosis). This was recognized more than seventy years ago, and since then there have been arguments both for and against using fluoride to help prevent tooth decay. At the concentration of one part per million (fluoride to water), there appears to be little evidence to suggest that fluoride has any side effects. This is the recommended concentration,[83] and it has been shown to effectively protect teeth from tooth decay. However, fluoride is potentially a very toxic element that is already present in our food, beverages, drugs, aerosols, nonstick pans, etc., as well as in fluoride tablets and toothpaste. We are surrounded, in a sense, by fluoride, and the real debate, as I see it, is how we can control and monitor the dosage our bodies are exposed to on a daily basis.

Fluorine

Fluorine is an extremely active element chemically, similar in many ways to chlorine. Both are very poisonous and readily combine with metals to form stable salts. Chlorine will combine with sodium to form sodium chloride, or common salt. Fluorine will behave in a similar way, forming a white sodium fluoride, which also tastes salty. When fluoride reacts with other materials, the resulting compound is often chemically stable. This reaction benefits our teeth by preventing them from dissolving in the acids produced in the dental plaque. But many are worried that[84] this stabilizing

---

83 Unicef—Official Position on Water Fluoridation: http://www.nofluoride.com/Unicef_fluor.htm
84 Connett, P. "Fluoride: A Statement of Concern." Jan 2000. http://www.fluoridealert.org/fluoride-statement.htm

influence may, if fluoride is present in our bodies in large amounts, have an adverse effect, locking up the vital minerals and enzymes necessary for good biological function. Do we want excess amounts of fluoride affecting the growth and development of our children's growing bones?

Dosage and the Effects on Teeth

The deciduous teeth, or baby teeth, do not appear to be substantially affected by fluoride during their formation. The evidence indicates[85] that little fluoride passes through the placental membrane; therefore, for those who wish to take fluoride supplements during pregnancy, there appears to be little advantage to either mother or baby.

Fluoride affects the permanent teeth, especially the enamel, and the dosage appears to be an all-important factor. Concentrations of up to one part per million appear to have few or no side effects on the enamel of the teeth.[86] In fact, many have observed that the enamel appears more pearly white and uniform in structure, and so it would seem that the fluoride not only makes the teeth more resistant to decay, but also makes them harder and cosmetically more pleasing.

There appears to be little leeway before mottling is evident on the teeth. Many authorities agree that one part per million is the approximate concentration when signs of fluorosis are unlikely to occur. At two parts per million, up to 10 percent of the teeth could show areas of brown stains or dull white opaque patches. At four parts per million, most growing teeth will be affected, with many badly stained and blotchy.[87]

---

85 Gedalia, I., et al. "Placental Transfer of Fluoride in the Human Fetus at Low and High F-Intake." J Dent Res. 1964:(43); 669.
86 CDC Statement on the 2006 National Research Council (NRC) Report on Fluoride in Drinking Water, Sept 24, 2008 http://www.cdc.gov/fluoridati on/safety/nrc_report.htm
87 (a) Hendrick, B., Ahmad, Z. "Excess Fluoride can hurt teeth, bones, I.Q." *Atlanta Journal-Constitution*, March 23, 2006

Some of the teeth may also have pitting of the surface enamel, and where there are brown stains, the enamel may be structurally weaker. The structural effects of fluorosis can penetrate the complete thickness of the tooth enamel, so intense brushing is unlikely to alter the color or staining of the damaged teeth.

If we are to look at the amount of dosage in perspective, one part per million means adding the equivalent of one tiny grain of salt to a large bucket of water. This can be described as a beneficial dose. What is of concern to me is that two tiny grains can have a harmful effect! We are all individuals, and no more so than in our dietary habits. Can we standardize how much water we consume, how much tea we drink, or how much fish we eat? Both tea and fish skin contain quite significant amounts of fluoride. If we are given a standard dose of any substance, do we react in a standardized way? The answer is no.

Fluoride and Tooth Decay

The popular impression is that fluoride protects the tooth by giving the enamel a protective and invisible shield. This is partly true, as the enamel is more resistant to attack from acids, just as paint helps protect a car from rusting. The fluoride does appear to concentrate on the surface of the enamel, thereby forming a less soluble layer. Fluoride will also influence the activity of the bacteria in the plaque. It does this in two ways: by interfering with the growth and behavior of the bacteria close to the surface of the tooth and by modifying the biochemical reactions that actually produce the acid.

Both of these factors demonstrate how fluoride is a powerful enzyme inhibitor. Fluoride also acts like a chemical buffer, reducing the activity of the acids and, in effect, neutralizing them. Another beneficial reaction in which fluoride contributes to the surface of the tooth is by encouraging the saliva to heal the enamel by laying down new minerals. This in turn reduces tooth sensitivity.

(b) Bryson, C. The Fluoride Deception. New York: Seven Stories Press, 2006 http://www.scribd.com/doc/11853971/the-fluoride-deceptionchristopher-bryson-398-3mb

It has been observed[88] that when fluoride has been taken during the formation of the teeth, their shape may be altered slightly.[89] The molars may have wider and shallower fissures and this has the advantage of reducing potential hiding places for bacteria and facilitating cleaning. Fluoride concentration in the teeth increases with age and this may be one of the reasons why the rate of tooth decay will often reduce as one becomes older.

Systemic Fluorides

Systemic means the inclusion of a substance into the whole body, and therefore systemic fluorides are those which, besides being incorporated into the tooth, can also be metabolized and incorporated into all the body tissues.

Fluoridation of Water Supplies

After many years of debate, in 1985 Parliament in Britain passed a bill enabling the water authorities to introduce fluoride into water supplies. Due to financial and technical difficulties, this does not mean that all areas of the country are fluoridated, but it does give the legal means whereby this can be achieved. Fluoridation has been introduced as a form of mass medication for the sole purpose of helping to prevent tooth decay. I believe it is a sad day when a nation has to be medicated because of a general failing in its diet and oral hygiene habits. There is also, of course, an ethical consideration: that of the right to choose.

Many people have fears that it is virtually impossible to control the total fluoride doses our bodies may receive, and this is magnified

---

88   European Commission: Scientific Committee on Consumer Product (SCCP)—"Opinion on the Safety of Fluorine Compounds in Oral Hygiene Product for Children Under the Age of 6 Years." 20 Sept 2005. http://ec.europa.eu/health/ph_risk/committees/04_sccp/docs/sccp_o_024.pdf

89   Van Sant, W. "Fluoride, a long time blessing, now a curse? A debate follows a warning by the ADA about giving babies fluoride water." June 2007. http://www.sptimes.com/2007/06/04/Tampabay/Fluoride__a_longtime_.shtml

by the inclusion of fluoride in our drinking water. Babies drink large amounts of fluid compared to their body weight, and should their nutrients be mixed and diluted with fluoridated water, this would be in addition to the existing concentration of fluoride already present in their food. If these foods have been produced or grown in an area of fluoridation, there must be concern about the amount of fluoride these tiny bodies are ingesting.

When food is processed using fluoridated water, the concentration of fluoride can increase dramatically. Gouda cheese, for instance, normally contains twenty-seven milligrams per kilogram of fluoride, but after processing with fluoridated water at one part per million, the levels of fluoride in the cheese can be increased by a factor of ten. Fruit and vegetables may also concentrate fluoride if there is abundance in the soil. In fluoridated areas, the watering of plants would be a source of this increase. Fluoride is also contained in some fertilizers and pesticides.

Tea contains fluoride, and many people can drink five or more cups a day. Reports of twenty cups a day are not uncommon. If the water to make the tea also contains fluoride, the daily intake may well exceed recommended safety levels.

The main disadvantage appears to be that by indiscriminately adding fluoride to the water, there can be no control on a chemical whose effect on the body we do not fully comprehend. The counterclaim is that fluoridation of our drinking water is a cost-effective way of reducing the level of tooth decay in the population. Figures of over 50 percent reduction in decay have been quoted from comparative surveys, and it would be of benefit to those members of our society whose priority does not lie in the care of their teeth. The debate continues!

If you do want to start young children on fluoride drops or tablets, seek professional advice from a dentist. In the United States, many medical doctors are now taking the responsibility for the supervision of fluoride administration. If the child is old enough, fluoride tablets are better sucked or chewed so that the fluoride can have an additional topical effect. There does seem to be considerable benefits regarding the reduction of tooth decay from the use of fluoride drops and tablets, but the disadvantage is that of maintaining a continuous daily intake throughout the period of tooth formation and eruption.

It is also important to keep fluoride tablets locked in the medicine cupboard, as an overdose can be very serious, as with any pharmaceutical drug. If such an unfortunate eventuality occurs, then you should obtain medical advice and treatment as soon as possible. Induce vomiting and give milk antacids or lime water to swallow.

The question "Should I give my children fluoride tablets?" is one I find difficult to answer. Fluoride will help protect the teeth, but I believe in the philosophy when prescribing drugs: *If in doubt, don't.* I am not convinced that enough research has been undertaken into the effects fluoride may have on our bones, organs, enzyme systems, and essential mineral reserves.

Both pro- and anti-fluoridation camps present statistics to enforce their arguments, but we all know how statistics can be presented to cast beneficial light on one's own point of view. Lack of fluoride is not the cause of tooth decay. Poor diet and poor oral hygiene are the most significant factors. It is ironic that the parents of children who are conscientious enough to enquire about fluoride administration are also the same parents who will ensure good supervision of home dental care and make sure their children have a low refined carbohydrate intake. Just the sort of parents whose children would most probably not require systemic fluoride! Fluoride is undeniably beneficial to our teeth, but why don't we concentrate on enriching the surface layers of the enamel rather than the whole body?

Topical Fluorides

This describes any method of fluoridation where the fluoride is applied directly onto the tooth and theoretically is not ingested and absorbed by the body.

Fluoride Toothpastes

One of the best methods of applying fluoride to the teeth is by using toothpaste. Nearly all (over 90 percent) of toothpastes sold in Europe and the United States contain a fluoride supplement. I am sure that fluoride toothpaste has played a significant role in reducing tooth decay. Different manufacturers use various systems to "deliver" fluoride to the surface enamel, and the concentration of fluoride in toothpaste can be as high as fifteen hundred parts per million. Thus, it is important to supervise children when they are brushing their teeth, if only to ensure that they do not swallow or eat the paste. Disturbing stories of children making toothpaste sandwiches and spearmint toothpaste drinks must be a warning to us all.

I believe that all the ingredients in the formulation of toothpaste should be clearly printed, and there should also be a large warning—DO NOT SWALLOW—clearly printed in the instructions (another possible use for toothpaste is to stick children's posters to their bedroom walls, as it apparently doesn't leave a mark, or so I'm told!).

Fluoride Gels

Many dentists, as part of a preventative regime, will apply a fairly concentrated (approximately 2 percent) solution, or gel, to the child's developing dentition. This would not normally take place before the age of six, as it is important that the patient is old enough to ensure that none of the fluoride is swallowed. This age will coincide with the eruption of the first molar teeth, and these are the teeth that often become heavily filled or lost due to early attacks of tooth decay.

If applied to these newly erupted teeth, fluoride uptake into the enamel appears to be good and offers protection at a time when it is most needed. Topical fluoride application can be of benefit at any age, but it is especially advantageous between the ages of six and fourteen years. There are adults who are particularly prone to tooth decay, and regular applications of topical fluoride, applied at the dental practice, can be included in a regime of dietary rehabilitation and oral hygiene techniques. In many dental practices, the hygienist often undertakes these valuable preventative measures.

Topical fluoride has been found to be of benefit to patients who suffer from sensitive teeth. The concentrated fluoride solution appears to provide a form of protection to the sensitive surface by blocking the microscopic pores where the nerves that transmit pain are stimulated.

Fluoride Mouth Rinses/Mouthwashes

Solutions can be obtained from the dentist, hygienist, or pharmacist in a less concentrated form for home use. However, these solutions must be treated as a potential poison and consequently should only be used with the explicit instructions of a dentist. They definitely are not suitable for young children. This is a useful method for regular home preventative treatment. Again, the same safety precautions should be adhered to with regard to home use and storage as with the drops and tablets.

In conclusion, fluoride is naturally present in the earth's crust, but experiments on animals[90] have shown that if they are totally deprived of fluoride, there appears to be no decline in their overall health. This would therefore signify that fluoride is not an essential nutrient. I therefore feel that introducing fluoride into our bodies is superfluous, and the emphasis should not be on how to increase our bodily intake, but on how to minimize it! Any method that delivers fluoride to the tooth surface should be encouraged.

---

90   (a) Pavlina, S. "What's the Deal With Fluoride?" July 19, 2005 http://www.stevepavlina.com/blog/2005/07/whats-the-deal-withfluoride/
(b) "The Health Dangers of Fluoride and Water Fluoridation." http://www.healthychoices.co.uk/fluoride.html

CHAPTER SEVEN

Gum Disease—What Lies Beneath?

Most of us do have some form of gum disease, and it's unlikely, unless we all change to a 100 percent *raw* whole food diet and can clean our teeth with 100 percent efficiency, that this situation will radically change. Remember that gum disease is a repeatable disease. A perfect diet and perfect cleaning once a week will do wonders, but the gum disease will come back if the regime is not continued. Good diet and hygiene need to become a lifestyle habit. Teeth can then remain solid in the jaw—even for a lifetime—something we all want ... and something that is certainly achievable.

Gum disease is the most common disease in the world, much more so than the common cold. In fact, there is undeniably some stage of the disease, however minor, in every single mouth. Most of the world's population has dental disease of some sort, and approximately 98 percent of that percentage is suffering from a clinically recognizable gum disease. It is the principal cause of tooth loss in people over the age of twenty-five globally.[91] If it cannot ever be entirely eradicated, as can tooth decay, it can be diminished largely by many of the same factors involved in the prevention of tooth decay—for example, good mouth hygiene, regular dental attendances, and, once again, diet.

Periodontal (gum) disease is an infection of the tissues that support the teeth. The gums support teeth. A tooth's root is anchored to its bone socket by fibers called periodontal ligaments. The gums do not attach to the teeth as firmly as one might think. A shallow V-shaped gap called the gum sulcus exists between the teeth and the gums. It is at this gap that periodontal disease occurs. If only the gums are

---

91 (a) American Dental Hygienists Association http://www.adha.org/oralhealth/adults.htm
(b) Statistics about Periodontitis http://www.wrongdiagnosis.com/p/periodontitis/stats.htm

involved, the disease is called gingivitis. If the tissues that hold the tooth to the jawbone are involved, it is called periodontitis.

Gum disease is much more destructive than tooth decay. Most decay in teeth can be halted, the teeth can be repaired, and the tooth can usually be saved. However, if gum disease is allowed to develop and progress, it threatens the foundation of the teeth and the bone that holds them in the jaw. Once bone loss occurs, the teeth become mobile, and ultimately they are likely to be lost.

Gums

The mouth is a break in the skin that covers and seals the entire body, making it a unique part of the human body. Skin stretches over the head, body, feet, and fingers, excluding only the eyes, and even the change from facial skin to the soft moist tissue inside the mouth is only a move from one type of skin to another. Skin stops our internal organs from falling out, and it prevents unwelcome microorganisms such as dirt and bacteria getting in.

When teeth are present in the mouth, there is a junction between the hard tooth and the nonmineralized skin, the gum. This junction is a break in the skin, which could be the reason that the gums are so vulnerable to disease. Because of that, the tooth-gum junction is, in a sense, a weak link in the overall design of the body coverage.

The principal function of the gums is to act as a protective covering over the bone holding the teeth, and to clasp tight against the teeth to prevent infection reaching the bone. Some people believe that the teeth are set into the gums, but in reality teeth are set into the bone, and the gums are merely a "skin."

Causes of Gum Disease

Bacterial Plaque

This sticky, colorless film constantly forms on our teeth and other tissues in the oral cavity. Plaque irritates the gums, causing them to become inflamed (red, tender, and swollen).

Brian Halvorsen, BDS, LDS RCS

Toxins produced by the bacteria in plaque irritate the gums. The toxins stimulate an inflammatory response in which the body in essence turns on itself and the tissues and bone that support the teeth are broken down and destroyed. Gums separate from the teeth, forming pockets (spaces between the teeth and gums) that become infected. As the disease progresses, the pockets deepen and more gum tissue and bone are destroyed.

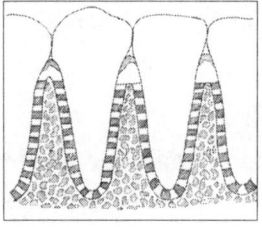

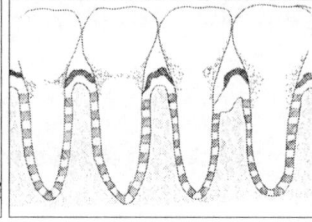

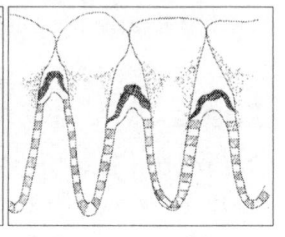

Illustrated by Caroline White

Copyright held by Brian Halvorsen

Credit: Illustrations by Caroline White, copyright Brian Halvorsen 2010.

Illustrated by Caroline White

Copyright held by Brian Halvorsen

Credit: Illustrations by Caroline White, copyright Brian Halvorsen 2010.

Illustrated by Caroline White

Copyright held by Brian Halvorsen

Credit: Illustrations by Caroline White, copyright Brian Halvorsen 2010

Fig. 13 (a)
Normal, Healthy Gums
Healthy gums and bone anchor teeth firmly in place.

Fig. 13 (b)
Periodontitis
Unremoved plaque hardens into calculus (tartar). As plaque and calculus continue to build up, the gums begin to recede (pull away) from the teeth, and pockets form between the teeth and gums.

Fig. 13 (c)
Advanced Periodontitis
The gums recede farther, destroying more bone and the periodontal ligament. Teeth—even healthy teeth—may become loose and need to be extracted.

Plaque that is not completely removed within forty-eight hours hardens into a rough deposit called tartar or calculus. Once tartar develops, the only way to remove it is by having the teeth professionally cleaned. Tartar below the gum line causes inflammation and infection. Because this process is often painless, a person may be unaware that a problem exists.

Holistic Causes of Gum Disease

Although plaque is the local cause of gum disease, there are also lifestyle and bodily health issues that can increase the likelihood of both the start and severity of periodontal disease.

Causes of Periodontal Disease[92]

The main cause of periodontal disease is bacterial plaque, a sticky, colorless film that constantly forms on your teeth. However, factors like the following also affect the health of your gums.

Smoking/Tobacco

As you probably already know, tobacco use is linked with many serious illnesses such as cancer, lung disease, and heart disease, as well as numerous other health problems. Tobacco users are also at increased risk for periodontal disease. In fact, recent studies have shown that tobacco use may be one of the most significant risk factors in the development and progression of periodontal disease.

Genetics

Research proves that up to 30 percent of the population may be genetically susceptible to gum disease. Despite aggressive oral care habits, these people may be six times more likely to develop

---

92 (a) "Causes of Gum Disease," American Academy of Periodontology. http://www.perio.org/consumer/gum-disease-causes.htm
(b) "Periodontal (Gum) Disease: Causes, Symptoms and Treatments," National Institute of Dental and Craniofacial Research, April 09. http://www.nidcr.nih.gov/OralHealth/Topics/GumDiseases/PeriodontalGumDisease.htm

periodontal disease. Identifying these people with a genetic test before they even show signs of the disease, and getting them into early interceptive treatment, may help them keep their teeth for a lifetime.

Pregnancy and Puberty

As a woman, you know that your health needs are unique. You know that brushing and flossing daily, a healthy diet, and regular exercise are all important to help you stay in shape. You also know that at specific times in your life, you need to take extra care of yourself. For example, when you mature and change, such as going through puberty or menopause, and when you have special health needs, such as menstruation or pregnancy, your body experiences hormonal changes. These changes can affect many of the tissues in your body, including your gums. Your gums can become sensitive and at times react strongly to the hormonal fluctuations. This may make you more susceptible to gum disease. Additionally, recent studies suggest that pregnant women with gum disease are seven times more likely to deliver preterm, low birth weight babies.

Stress

As you probably already know, stress is linked to many serious conditions such as hypertension, cancer, and numerous other health problems. What you may not know, though, is that stress is also a risk factor for periodontal disease. Research demonstrates that stress can make it more difficult for the body to fight off infection, including periodontal disease.

Medications

Some drugs, such as oral contraceptives, antidepressants, and certain heart medicines, can affect your oral health. Just as you notify your pharmacist and other health care providers of all medicines you are taking and any changes in your overall health, you should also inform your dental care provider.

Clenching or Grinding Your Teeth

Has anyone ever told you that you grind your teeth at night? Is your jaw sore from clenching your teeth when you're taking a test or solving a problem at work? Clenching or grinding your teeth can put excess force on the supporting tissues of the teeth and could speed up the rate at which these periodontal tissues are destroyed.

Diabetes

Diabetes is a disease that causes altered levels of sugar in the blood. Diabetes develops from either a deficiency in insulin production (a hormone that is the key component in the body's ability to use blood sugars) or from the body's inability to use insulin correctly. According to the American Diabetes Association, approximately sixteen million Americans have diabetes; however, more than half have not been diagnosed with this disease. If you are diabetic, you are at higher risk for developing infections, including periodontal diseases. These infections can impair the ability to process and/or utilize insulin, which may cause your diabetes to be more difficult to control and your infection to be more severe than that of a nondiabetic.

Poor Nutrition

As you may already know, a diet low in important nutrients can compromise the body's immune system and make it harder for the body to fight off infection. Because periodontal disease is a serious infection, poor nutrition can worsen the condition of your gums.

Other Systemic Diseases

Diseases that interfere with the body's immune system may worsen the condition of the gums.

Types of Periodontal Disease

There are many forms of periodontal disease. The most common ones include the following:

Gingivitis

This is the mildest form of periodontal disease. It causes the gums to become red, swollen, and bleed easily. There is usually little or no discomfort at this stage. Gingivitis is reversible with professional treatment and good home care.

Acute Gum Disease

Most gum disease is chronic, meaning that it can rumble on slowly before showing any clinical symptoms. However, children from puberty onward, from about twelve to twenty years, can develop an acute, or rapidly progressing, condition known as juvenile periodontitis. This is associated with periods of severe gum infection and areas of severe bone loss around the teeth. It is normally treated with mouthwashes and intensive gum therapy, but it is a classic instance of where the whole person should be considered. As far as nutrition is concerned, this can be a bad age and also a time of great stress, with pressures at school, exams coming around with unremitting regularity, and the emotional traumas and physical changes of puberty. Comparatively little research has been undertaken on these aspects, despite the fact that there would seem to be a logical association.

Another stress-related condition is AUG (acute ulcerative gingivitis)—"Vincent's infection" or "trench mouth." The gums are painful, red, and bleeding. Ulcers and pus can also be present. AUG develops rapidly, and some think it is contagious because it can affect people in groups. Men in the trenches of World War I suffered it because of the triple combination of poor diet, bad hygiene, and stress. Nowadays it afflicts people who may have a chronic gum condition and become stressed, especially where there are severe emotional strains. Antibiotics like metronidazole and penicillins can be very useful, followed by oral hygiene and treatment from the hygienist.

Chronic Gum Disease

If left untreated, gingivitis can lead to chronic gum disease or periodontitis. The bone supporting the teeth shrinks from the root, often accompanied by swollen gums. The resultant pockets make cleaning the teeth more difficult, in turn leading to more gum disease. This then leads to a cycle of deterioration that is characterized by periods of chronic and acute phases of the disease. Recognized as the most frequently occurring form of periodontitis, it is age related.

Diagnosing Gum Disease

A dentist's confirmation and advice should always be sought as soon as any signs of gum disease manifest themselves. Fear often prevents a dental consultation, but it must be remembered that the sooner treatment is started, the sooner the disease process can be halted. If left, it can only deteriorate, and subsequent treatment, discomfort, and eventual health of the mouth will be much worse. Never be afraid to go to the dentist.

The Signs of Gum Disease

Bleeding Gums

Do your gums bleed? Any bleeding indicates the beginnings of gum disease, and this can occur when brushing, when eating, or with gentle probing. Obviously, an accidental knock on the gums, which splits the skin, will cause bleeding, but the gums should be firm enough to withstand quite rigorous brushing without blood being drawn.

As soon as any blood is seen on the brush (provided this hasn't been caused by too harsh brushing), in the spat-out saliva/toothpaste, or on the gum itself, this means that there is gum disease (gingivitis) present. Often, bleeding from the gums is so common and becomes so habitual that most people don't worry about it. It's in these early stages that the owner of the gums can do the most to alleviate and halt the process, so any bleeding should never be ignored.

The adage "Ignore it and it'll go away" could not be more wrong when considering gum disease, or, with justification, it could be reinterpreted as "Ignore bleeding from the gums and your teeth will go away." For that initial bleeding of gingivitis or inflammation of the gum can lead very swiftly to the more severe form of gum disease, when bone loss is involved (periodontitis) and where tooth loss may become inevitable.

In these early disease stages, the mouth shows some of its unique properties. It's different from the rest of the body in that it's rare for an infection to cause open bleeding. If you get an infection elsewhere, there will probably be pus and fluid. In the gums, though, blood is the first sign, and if pus does occur, this means the disease is advanced. Also, the action demanded by bleeding in the mouth is quite different from that accorded to bleeding elsewhere in the body.

If you have a cut on the hand or leg, or even a bleeding lip, the last thing you would want to do is to brush it, poke it, and continually wash it. You would want the blood to clot. But in the mouth, if you have bleeding, the last thing you want to do is leave it alone!

In order to stop bleeding of the gums, the only answer is to brush more, irrigate more, and generally pay much more attention to the site of the bleeding. Although there may be more bleeding at first in response to careful and thorough brushing, *the more you brush and irrigate, the less the gum will bleed,* and the quicker it will return to normal, healthy tissue.

It's a vicious circle; we are conditioned by our instinctive reactions to bleeding elsewhere in the body. We don't brush our teeth because it makes the gums bleed, but the gums are bleeding because the teeth are not being brushed! To prevent gum disease, the teeth, in theory, need only be thoroughly brushed once a day, but once disease is present, the teeth and gums need to be brushed more often.

Red and Swollen Gums

This is a definite sign of acute gum disease (gingivitis), along with bleeding. Gums will change to red from their normal pink color, and there will be swelling, especially between the teeth, and tenderness. Any alteration in the appearance, color, or size of gums should be taken seriously, and a dentist's advice should be sought.

Unpleasant Taste or Bad Breath

Blood and infection may cause a bad taste from the gums. It may also be food debris stagnating on the gum or in the gum crevices. This is not an entirely reliable sign because the more a taste is present, the less the taste buds will recognize it as alien. As with bad breath, individuals may become quickly accustomed to it, for the same reason. Every dentist will be able to differentiate the characteristic smell of gum disease from bad breath food stagnation, tummy upsets, or sinus infections. This odor is associated with advanced gum disease, and it smells, frankly, of putrefaction.

Receding gums

Disease causes the gums to shrink away from the crowns of the teeth, and it will expose the roots. With less support from the gums, the teeth will be less secure. Age, as mentioned already, can cause gum recession not directly associated with gum disease. This is why older people are said to be "long in the tooth," for gum recession does inevitably make the teeth look longer. Gums can also shrink back through excessive tooth brushing. Age-related gum recession is regarded as "normal wear and tear," but does vary from person to person. Your dentist will explain on an individual basis why this is happening, and if the recession of the gum can be prevented.

Discomfort and pain

Gum disease does not usually cause discomfort, but when pain occurs, it normally means there is an active infection. This occurs in acute attacks or if the act of brushing more thoroughly starts an inflammation in a part of the mouth that has a preexisting gum condition. Brushing can cause discomfort or pain, and a distinct aching and itching can also be symptoms. This is not an excuse to stop brushing! Abscesses can be caused by gum disease and will obviously cause pain. They occur on the side of teeth rather than at the tip of the root, when the infected contents of the deepened gum pocket cannot escape into the mouth. Abscesses caused by periodontitis can rapidly damage the supporting bone around the affected tooth.

Change of Bite

If there is a change in the way that your teeth come together, this can mean that the teeth are starting to move because of bone loss due to gum disease. It is not the only cause, as clenching and problems with the jaw joints can also make the teeth feel as if they are not meeting properly.

Pus

Pus is the sign of a severe infection in any part of the body, and particularly in the mouth. Dental advice must be sought as soon as possible and treatment instituted immediately. It can show as a yellow color between the teeth, and it can come out of the gums when you press on them.

Loose or Separating Permanent Teeth

Unless you are between six and twelve, when you might expect to have loose teeth, any mobility may be caused by gum disease. This is when the foundation bone has been severely eroded, and inflammation may extend over most of the root of the tooth. Once this extends around the end of the root, the tooth will fall out. If the teeth are also separating, however slightly, it means that they're actually drifting apart as well as loosening. It is very distressing on front teeth, where it's commonly seen as spreading and splaying of the incisors.

Another common sign of gum disease is when one incisor appears to grow longer than the other. The body is almost starting to reject the teeth, and it doesn't want them there anymore. This is severe gum disease and purely conventional treatment; even scaling every six weeks will not be truly effective. Your dentist may refer you to a gum specialist, referred to as a periodontist.

The Progress of Gum Disease

Warning Signs, Stages of Gum Disease

1. Bleeding gums — Early sign
2. Red, swollen, or tender gums — Early sign in most cases
3. Bad breath and bad taste — Early or advanced
4. Receding gums — Early or advanced
5. Discomfort and pain — Usually advanced
6. Change of bite — Advanced
7. Change in partial denture fit — Advanced
8. Pus — Bad advanced
9. Loose or separating teeth — Severe advanced

Warning: Gum disease is associated with increased cancer risk.

In a study of more than forty-eight thousand men who were studied over a period of more than seventeen years[93]—after adjustment for known risk factors including smoking and dietary factors—participants with a history of gum disease had a 14 percent higher risk of cancer compared with those with no history of gum disease. The most common cancers were colorectal, melanoma, lung, bladder, and advanced prostate cancer.

"Periodontal disease might be a marker of a susceptible immune system or might directly affect cancer risk."[94]

Advice: Please visit your dentist and hygienist regularly.

Additional Mouth Conditions

Ulcers or sores can develop from viruses such as herpes, both inside and outside the mouth. Other infections such as candida can cause soreness and irritation. Some drugs can cause a sensitivity reaction in the mouth, with swelling, soreness, and ulcers. The eruption of the wisdom teeth can cause inflammation and ultimate infection at the back of the mouth.

Mouth ulcers are very common, occurring in some 40 to 50 percent of the population.[95] They are painful, worrying in that it is a breakdown in the skin for no apparent reason, and they can and do recur. Nutritional deficiencies are the main cause. Giving certain vitamins can reduce the amount of ulceration and frequency. Some practitioners (including myself) have used mega doses of vitamin C and zinc supplementation to reduce the frequency of mouth ulcers.[96]

---

93   (a) US health professionals who started at Harvard in 1986
     (b) *Lancet Oncology*. Volume 9
94   (a) *Lancet Oncology*. Volume 9
     (b) Report published in British Dental Journal Vol. 204, June 2008
95   (a) "Mouth Ulcer," NHS Choices http://www.nhs.uk/conditions/mouth-ulcer/Pages/Introduction.aspx
     (b) "Aphthous Mouth Ulcers, Patient UK." http://www.patient.co.uk/showdoc/23068855/
96   (a) "Therapy of Mouth Ulcer." http://www.dhyansanjivani.org/therapy_mouth.asp

A dentist should be consulted if any mouth condition gives concern. Later I will discuss mouth cancer.

A Review of Nutrition's Impact on Gum Disease

Remember that gum disease relates to living tissue, and therein lies a major difference from tooth decay. It could be argued that a tooth is living, but in fact the surface layers are inert, with no nerve endings or blood supply. Gum disease can begin so much more rapidly than tooth decay. Although an acidic attack on a tooth can begin within minutes, the tooth will not suffer clinical damage for months. In twenty-four hours, though, because of poor resistance, the initial stages of gum disease can become quite severe.

I have listed the causes of gum disease, and I am certain that poor nutrition must be the major one. Because host resistance to disease is affected by health, and health is affected by nutrition, gum disease must have a relationship to nutrition. Although there was an upsurge of interest in nutrition and dental health in the twenties and thirties, since then the subject has not been explored in any great depth, either in research or in the textbooks.

The emphasis has been on the treatment of disease rather than on the causes, and although treatment is obviously vital, it's a rather blinkered situation. Why is dental disease more prevalent now, despite these advances in science and all these treatments? Could this be due to faulty nutrition? Could it also be due to environmental stresses, which are more severe now than fifty years ago, as with personal lifestyle stresses? Researchers need to take into account the people who suffer from disease, and by looking at them holistically, proper clinical evaluations can be made.

Most diseases are multifactorial in origin; they can rarely be attributed to one cause alone. This is why only a percentage of those who smoke contract lung cancer. So, if environmental stresses cannot be altered, and personal emotional stresses are difficult to counteract, a good diet would seem to be a major way in which

---

(b) "Mouth Ulcers, Bleeding Gums, Bad Breath." http://www.sunspirit.com.au/mouth_ulcers_bad_breath.htm

body resistance to disease can be boosted. A good whole food diet, which will improve general health, will undoubtedly help in the fight against gum disease. Rather than just accept poor nutrition as a cause of disease, let's use good nutrition as a weapon to fight it.

Dietary Supplements

It is believed that certain dietary supplements help in the fight against gum disease. Vitamin C, for instance, prevented scurvy, the primary symptoms of which were bleeding gums. Increased intake of vitamin C is known to help regenerate tissue and boost the immune system. For many years, I have recommended one thousand milligrams of vitamin C as a minimum daily dose for my patients who are suffering from gum disease.

A case example: A middle-aged woman on steroid medication was suffering from severe mouth ulceration and sore gums. Her medical doctor recommended five hundred milligrams of vitamin C daily. The patient responded well, but within two months, ulcers reappeared. I recommended taking one thousand milligrams of timed-release vitamin C daily, and her gums and ulcers dramatically improved. When she lowered the dose of vitamin C to five hundred milligrams, symptoms returned. I concluded that for this patient she needed at least one thousand milligrams of vitamin C daily to remain symptomless (orally).

Supplementation of our diet is becoming increasingly important in our stressful world. Always seek the advice of a nutritional expert to prescribe the correct nutrition program, as we are all individuals.

So, if we can't be perfect, we should work toward slowing down the progress of the disease and boosting our immune system. In this way, we might still have minor signs of gum disease, but we will not be troubled by it. Globally, the World Health Organization (WHO) states that "oral health means much more than healthy teeth—oral health is integral to general health." Increasingly research is showing[97] links between gum disease, heart disease, pancreatic

---

97 (a) "Gum Disease Links to Heart Disease and Stroke." http://www.perio.org/consumer/mbc.heart.htm

cancer, diabetes, stroke, osteoporosis, and premature births. Is gum disease a symptom of a diseased body, or vice versa?

Incidentally, smoking diminishes vitamin C in the body. Many gum specialists (periodontists) will not treat patients if they continue smoking. Another readily available supplement, coenzyme Q10, has also been shown[98] to boost the immune system, and Q10 has been shown to reduce gum inflammation in clinical trials.

The Role of the Dentist

In diagnosing gum disease and treating it, the dentist plays a pivotal role. By preventing gum disease, he will not only be saving teeth, but also improving the general health of his patient.

Sixty years ago, the dreaded word "pyorrhea," an old-fashioned word for periodontitis, would have meant extraction of some, if not all, of the teeth. Gum disease can now be halted, and teeth can be saved. I cannot emphasize enough how important it is for a dentist to be consulted regularly, and as soon as any signs of the disease become apparent.

Although home brushing can often cope with the first signs of bleeding gums, one should make her dentist aware of the situation. He or his team can advise on brushing. Gums can literally heal within hours; a soft brush and a thorough and careful brushing will remove the first layers of plaque, and the gums can begin the healing process. Today there are many oral hygiene aids. The dentist and his team can tailor these tools to suit the individual requirements for the patient.

(b) "Gum Disease Link to Cancer Risk," 26 May 2008, Lancet KR 200, BBC News, http://news.bbc.co.uk/1/hi/health/7416672.stm

(c) "Study finds New Evidence of Periodontal Disease Leading to Gestational Diabetes." 6 April 2009. http://www.medicalnewstoday.com/arti cles/145159.php

98   "Coenzyme Q10," University of Maryland Medical Center http://www.umm.edu/altmed/articles/coenzyme-q10-000295.htm

CHAPTER EIGHT

Oral Hygiene: Ignore Your Teeth and Gums—and They Will Go Away!

Oral hygiene is the most direct way to remove plaque. I don't believe that anyone can ever guarantee to be 100 percent efficient, but any cleaning will help diminish the attacks by plaque. So why not aim to do the very best possible in the cause of a healthy mouth and sound teeth and gums. It may be a chore, but the amount of time you spend every day keeping your mouth clean is one of the best investments you can make for health and lasting good looks of your teeth. Remember, by removing the plaque that causes gum disease, you will also remove the plaque that causes tooth decay!

Tooth Brushing

This is the key to plaque control, for plaque cannot be washed off the teeth, it must be abraded or brushed off. Brushing with a clean toothbrush—without any toothpaste—would also be the most natural process of cleaning your teeth. It does not introduce any chemicals, nor upset the balance of the oral flora, and it does not involve the ingestion of anything that might be harmful. Brushing literally breaks down any established plaque and disorganizes it. If you brush several times a day, plaque will not be given the chance to settle anywhere, and thus you will be severely impeding the progress of both tooth decay and gum disease.

The number of times you should brush per day depends on how effective your technique is. To be safe, to prevent tooth decay, you should brush after every meal. To prevent the possibility of plaque reacting with sugars, teeth should be brushed free of plaque before a meal, thereby eliminating the presence of plaque and its potential interaction with any sugars. For most people, twice a day, after breakfast and before going to bed, seems to be the norm.

Great Teeth for Life

Once gum disease has developed, in however minor a form, more frequent brushing is vital to get rid of accumulated plaque and bring the gums back to health. The action of brushing the gums, not just the teeth, appears to improve the health of the gums. The friction stimulates the blood supply and hardens the gum tissue.

How to Brush Your Teeth

Home brushing is a major factor in plaque control, but it is at the dental inspection or visit to the hygienist that the brushing technique can be assessed. A faulty technique can be corrected, or a better one advised.

We are creatures of habit—and tooth brushing is not an exception. When the dentist/hygienist points out areas of the mouth that are habitually missed, then shows an improved method of cleaning those areas, this is prevention in practice. Over time, a patient's oral hygiene improves, and the threat of avoidable mouth disease lessens.

This has a dual benefit. It shows the patient what can be done, often at no more than the cost of a toothbrush, and builds a trusting and caring relationship with the dentist and hygienist. When time is spent giving instructions on how to brush, patients say their mouths feel much cleaner and healthier thereafter. Feedback like this is vital for a dentist, and it is fundamental for the relationship between dentist and patient. If the dentist has managed to improve the situation, even in a minor way, the patient will feel better and more positive about his mouth and teeth, knowing he can do so much more for himself.

Styles of brushing vary, and they tend to go through fashions. At one time, it was up and down, then it was from side to side ... and it's no wonder that people get confused. However, as I've emphasized throughout the book, any method will be unique to the individual. Everybody has teeth and jaws of different shapes and sizes, so the ideal cleaning techniques will differ. This is where individual tuition is important. This is the role of the dentist and his team—the dental health educator, the dental therapist and the dental hygienist—to provide each patient with his own "personal trainer" in oral health.

The present technique recommended by the profession is a small rotary action, in which the gum and tooth are massaged together, with the brush held at an angle of about forty-five degrees to the gum/tooth junction. Cover only two or three teeth at a time so that you don't miss any. The movement should be firm but not too hard; too vigorous brushing can actually damage the tooth enamel and can make the gums shrink back, exposing the cementum and dentin. The final step is to rinse the mouth out thoroughly with water.

You should try to brush your teeth in front of a mirror so that you can see what you are doing, and that the brush is going where it ought to go. Many recommend brushing for two minutes. Personally, I believe that the important issue is the effective removal of the dental plaque, not how long it takes or what style of toothbrush is being used.

Toothbrushes

The toothbrush seems to have its origins in the chewing sticks of Babylonia, as early as 3500 BC. Ancient Greek and Roman literature discusses the use of toothpicks, which were used to keep the mouth clean, although they were only mentioned, with no further description given. Over the years, the toothpick evolved into a chew stick, which was the size of a pencil.

Records from China around 1600 BC show that one end was chewed until it became brushlike; the other end was pointed and used as a toothpick. The twigs used for this purpose were from aromatic trees and therefore freshened the mouth as well as cleaned it.

The first bristled toothbrush also originated from China at around the same time and was brought back to Europe by traders. It was made from hairs from the neck of the Siberian wild boar, which were fixed to a bamboo or bone handle. In Europe, where few people brushed their teeth, wild boar hairs were too stiff and made the gums bleed, so horsehair, which was softer, was used instead. It was still more customary in Europe to use a toothpick made of a goose feather, silver, or copper after meals.[99]

In the eighteenth century, the invention of the modern toothbrush was attributed to William Addis, a stationer whose name became attached to the household brush company. In hiding after the Gordon Riots (a predominantly Protestant uprising against the Papist Act of 1778, which had in turn been aimed at removing restrictions against Catholics) in London, England, in 1780, Addis hid in a slaughterhouse, where he whiled away the hours by carving bone. He then had the brilliant idea of boring small holes in one end of a bone handle and inserting horsehair into them. This, then, was the inauspicious origin of the first modern toothbrush! In 1857, America entered the toothbrush market when H. N. Wadsworth was awarded the first patent in America for their production. In 1937, Dupont laboratories invented nylon in the United States. Nylon was first used as the bristles in their toothbrush in 1938: Dr. West's "miracle" toothbrush with nylon bristles. Interestingly it wasn't until WWII that the concept of brushing teeth caught on in the States, partly because it was compulsory for American soldiers to clean their teeth regularly!

Since then, the toothbrush has been refined and modified, with handles of celluloid, then plastic, with bristles of natural bristle or nylon. The industry has flourished. Britain is apparently one of the top three consumers of toothbrushes per capita in the world, but it is also a virtually static consumption. Despite recommendations from dentists that brushes should be replaced every two to three months at the longest, the average adult buys only 1.25 brushes per year, around fifty-six million brushes in 1984. The year 2009 saw slightly higher annual sales but no significant changes in toothbrush sales per capita per year since 1984.[100]

---

99 Toothbrush History. http://www.toothbrushexpress.com/html/toothbrush_history.html
100 "Report on UK Toothbrushes Market, Research, Trends, Analysis," 2004. http://www.the-infoshop.com/study/mt19665_toothbrushes.html

Again, people should consult their dentists and hygienists about the type of brush to use, for individual instruction is necessary. There are literally about a hundred different types of toothbrush designs on the market, with varying sizes, types of bristles, lengths of handles ... all of which can influence how well the toothbrush is used. In general, though, the surround of the head, the part in which the bristles are set, should be smooth and rounded so that nothing can jar against tissues in the mouth, and the head itself should be fairly small. With a large head, you could probably sweep over about four teeth at a time, missing small areas. With a small head, you can more painstakingly concentrate on each tooth.

The bristles should be made of nylon, not natural bristle. Natural bristle has larger filaments than nylon, and the ends are cut during the manufacturing process. If the massaging method of cleaning is used with natural bristles, the sharp cut-off ends of these bristles can microscopically cut the gums. Nylon filaments have rounded and polished ends. They are also designed specifically to be soft enough to bend and flex into the two-millimeter gum crevice of theoretical perfect health. Toothbrush filaments should be hard enough to remove plaque but soft enough so that they won't damage the gum. Hard brushes are unnecessary. The dentist or hygienist will be able to advise on the number of bristle rows needed on the brush head. This again relates to the size of mouth and teeth.

Many manufacturers are now designing their toothbrush handles with heads of flexi-plastic. This means that the user can actually bend and modify the head to improve efficiency. This idea could do away with any need to buy different brushes for different jobs.

Take care of your brush, and it will last longer. Don't use warm water to dampen it, as this will soften the nylon and may permanently distort it. Try not to use water that is too cold either, as this could set your teeth on edge. Wash the brush after use to get rid of any debris, and knock it lightly against the side of the basin to get rid of excess water. Store it upright in a wall-hung tray preferably, so that it can drain properly.

Do try to change your brush several times a year. Normally I would say every month or six weeks, but it varies from person to person.

When the bristles start to splay, they will not reach into the gum crevice, so that is the time for a change. If you brush your teeth as instructed by the dentist, and you find a brush splays after about a week or so, it might be worth complaining to the manufacturer or trying out another brand to see if that lasts any longer.

Electric Toothbrushes

The electric toothbrush uses electric power to move the brush head, normally in an oscillating pattern, though electric toothbrushes are often called "rotary" toothbrushes.

In the late 1800s in the United States, a notorious quack named Dr. Scott claimed to invent an "electric" toothbrush. However, unlike actual electric bristle brushes, Dr. Scott's brush merely sent a strong electrical current through the brush to its user. The shock was apparently (according to lore of the time) supposed to "promote good health."[101]

Although a true electric toothbrush was first conceived in 1954 and sold in 1956 in Switzerland, the Broxodent was a rotating electric toothbrush introduced by Squibb Pharmaceutical at the centennial of the American Dental Association in 1960. These were initially created for patients with limited manual dexterity, as well as those with orthodontic appliances.

Effectiveness

According to the marketing campaigns, electric toothbrushes are more efficient than their manual variants, but research doesn't seem to prove this.

Independent research finds that most electric toothbrushes are no more effective than the manual variety. The exception is the "rotation-oscillation" models, where the small round head rotates in one direction, then reverses direction, but even these perform only marginally better than a regular manual brush. The research

---

[101] "Electric Toothbrush History." http://en.wikipedia.org/wiki/Electric_toothbrush

indicates that the way the brushing is performed is of higher importance than the choice of brush.[102]

For people who, for various reasons, have problems with their manual dexterity (i.e., people with arthritis and the elderly), electric brushes can be, and often are, essential.

If the brusher enjoys brushing with an electric toothbrush, I have often seen a significant improvement in her oral hygiene. I believe the simple electric toothbrush has now become a vital part in the armory in combating dental disease.

Thorough brushing is all that is needed for healthy teeth and gums, for toothpaste isn't strictly necessary, so there's no excuse not to carry a brush with you at all times, whether in your pocket, briefcase, or handbag. Small fold-up travelling brushes are also available. Airlines are supplying toothbrushes on long-haul flights—good for them! I have also seen machines that dispense disposable brushes already pasted. Wouldn't it be something if toothbrush dispensers were in competition with condoms, etc., in the restrooms of hotels and restaurants?

Toothpaste

As long ago as 5000 BC, the Egyptians were making a tooth powder consisting of powdered ashes of ox hooves, myrrh, powdered and burnt eggshells, and pumice. There are directions about relative quantities that should be mixed, but no instructions are available about how this powder was used. It is assumed that it was rubbed onto the teeth using the fingers, as the tooth stick—the forerunner to the toothbrush—was not in use at that time.

The Greeks, and then the Romans, improved the recipes for toothpaste by adding abrasives such as crushed bones and oyster shells, which were used to clean debris from teeth. The Romans added powdered charcoal, powdered bark, and more flavoring agents to improve the breath.

---

102 "Thumbs Down for Electric Toothbrush," BBC News, Health, 21 January 2003. http://news.bbc.co.uk/1/hi/health/2679175.stm

Great Teeth for Life

Few records then relate to the existence of toothpaste or powder until around 1000 AD, when the Persians wrote to advise their people to be wary of the dangers of using hard abrasives as toothpowders. They recommended that people use burnt hart's horn, the burnt shells of snails, and burnt gypsum. Other Persian recipes involved dried animal parts, herbs, honey, and minerals. One recipe to strengthen teeth includes green lead, verdigris, incense, honey, and powdered flint.[103]

There is then another huge gap in the history of toothpaste until the eighteenth century, when toothpowder, or dentifrice, became available in Britain. Doctors and dentists developed these powders and chemists, and they included substances abrasive to teeth, such as brick dust, crushed china, earthenware, and cuttlefish. Bicarbonate of soda was used as the basis for most toothpowders, and some contained other ingredients that would not be considered appropriate today, such as sugar. Borax powder was added at the end of the eighteenth century to produce a favorable foaming effect. The rich applied toothpowder with a brush. The poor cleaned their teeth with bicarbonate of soda, using their fingers.

Glycerin was added early in the nineteenth century to make the powders into a paste and thereby more palatable.

Also introduced at this time was strontium, which serves to strengthen teeth and reduce sensitivity. A dentist called Peabody became the first person to add soap to toothpowder in 1824, and John Harris added chalk in the 1850s.

In 1873, toothpaste was first mass-produced. It was in a jar, and it smelled good for the first time, as now peppermint was added for flavor. In 1892, Dr. Washington Sheffield of Connecticut was the first to put toothpaste into a collapsible tube: Dr. Sheffield's Creme Dentifrice. Sheffield's company was to become Colgate.

---

103 "The History of Teeth Cleaning," BBC Home. http://www.bbc.co.uk/dna/h2g2/A2818686

Brian Halvorsen, BDS, LDS RCS

Components of Today's Toothpaste

The formulation of a typical toothpaste is described in the following table:

Component	Function	Examples	% (w/w)
Polishing Agent	Abrasive that helps in the removal of plaque and extrinsic tooth stain without scratching the tooth enamel or dentin	Calcium carbonate, hydrated silicas, dicalcium phosphate, alumina, glycerin, sorbitol	15–50
Humectant	Holds water in the toothpaste: stops 'plugging' in the nozzle, helps dissolve some of the other ingredients, provides gloss to the paste, and can impart sweetness	Glycerin, sorbitol	30–60
Gum Thickeners	Controls consistency, improving flow of the toothpaste onto the brush and dispersion in the mouth. Gums also bind the solid and liquid together to maintain the integrity of the paste	Sodium carboxymethyllcellulose carrageenan, xanthan	0.5–2.0
Other Thickeners	Colloidal or particulate thickeners are used in addition to gums in many formulations to give more 'body' and gel-like character to toothpastes, particularly if low concentrations of the (solid) abrasives are used	Laponite synthetic clay, colloidal hydrated silicas	0–15
Foaming Agent	Detergent: provides foam that eases the removal of food debris and improves dispersion in the mouth	Sodium laurylsulphate (SLS), sodiummethylcocoyl taurate (in Macleans Sensitive)	0.5–2.0
Component Flavor System	Very important from the consumer's point of view: makes the product pleasant to use and leaves a fresh taste in the mouth	Peppermint and spearmint (most common in mass market), sodium saccharin, menthol, aniseed, lemon oil, eucalyptus	0.3–1.6

Primary Ingredients	Protect against tooth decay, gum disease, and tartar, and treat sensitivity	Very diverse, e.g., fluoride systems (sodium fluoride), sodium monofluorophosphate, antimicrobials (triclosan, zinc citrate), tartar agents (sodium and potassium pyrophosphates), sensitivity agents (potassium nitrate and strontium acetate), stain removal agent (sodium tripolyphosphate)	0.2–8
Preservatives	To preserve the product from microbiological attack during consumer use	Sodium propyl paraben, sodium methyl paraben, potassium sorbate, benzoic acid	0.05–0.1
Coloring	Important for visual aspect	Various dyes	Trace amounts
Water	Solubilise and carry some of the active ingredients, and make up the liquid phase of the toothpaste	Processed water, in some cases treated to remove minerals	To 100%

What's in Your Toothpaste?

Although toothpaste is not ingested, and should not be, holistic dentists feel that the ingredients of toothpaste should be listed on packaging, as food manufacturers are obliged to do so. It's not a food, but it is sold and bought as one, in a sense. I will disclose a much more detailed list of ingredients.

As far as I know, this is the first time such a comprehensive list of ingredients of "normal" toothpaste has ever been published.

Primary Ingredients

Baking Soda/Bicarbonate of Soda ($NaHCO_3$):

Baking soda has the potential to modify the pH of plaque, and possibly the virulence of the bacteria that cause decay. It may also interfere with plaque metabolism and reduce acid production. Baking soda has a distinctive flavor, perceived by the consumer to give a cleaner and fresher mouth.

Calcium Glycerophosphate (CaGP):

CaGP can increase the amount of fluoride that is absorbed into the enamel and helps strengthen the enamel. Having CaGP present in the toothpaste can increase the amount of calcium and phosphate that is available for the remineralisation of enamel. In a caries clinical trial, toothpaste with 0.13 percent CaGP was more effective than toothpaste with just fluoride present.

Cetylpyridinium Chloride (CPC):

CPC is a guarternary ammonium compound. Quaternary ammonium compounds are cationic agents capable of reducing surface tension. CPC adsorbs to the surface of bacterial cells and disrupts the cell membrane by affecting the surface tension. CPC is a broad-spectrum antimicrobial that can perform better than chlorhexidine when it is tested in vitro, but is not as effective in practice against plaque. The reason for this is that CPC is cleared more quickly from the mouth, whereas chlorhexidine salts are retained. It has also been suggested that CPC loses some of its potency when it is bound to a surface such as tooth enamel. As with chlorhexidine salts, CPC has been reported to stain the teeth, but not at the 0.1 percent levels used in some SB products. CPC is extremely difficult to formulate as an effective toothpaste.

Calcium Carbonate/Chalk ($CaCO_3$):

Calcium carbonate has abrasive/cleaning properties that ensure removal of plaque, food debris, and extrinsic stain. It also neutralizes the acids that are produced by plaque.

Chlorhexidine Salts (Gluconates, Acetates and Chlorides):

Chlorhexidine is a member of the bis-biguanide family. The bis-biguanides constitute a group of antimicrobial agents that have been used as broad-spectrum antiseptics since 1953. These compounds offer the advantage of combining antibacterial properties with low toxicity as they are poorly absorbed through the lining of the mouth or in the gastrointestinal tract. Chlorhexidine salts are effective against a wide variety of bacteria. Indeed, they are regarded as being the "gold standard" for effectiveness against plaque and gingivitis, and they have been reported to inhibit plaque acid production. Chlorhexidine salts have the ability to bind to cell membranes and alter membrane permeability. This results in leakage of intracellular components and the precipitation and coagulation of cycoplasmic contents of the bacterial cell. A key property of chlorhexidine salts that separates them from other antimicrobials is their ability to bind to the surfaces of the oral cavity and be released slowly, prolonging the duration of action. This binding power also creates an ability to bind tannin and other staining agents to the teeth, although a dentist or dental hygienist can remove these stains.

The most widely used chlorhexidine salt is chlorhexidine gluconate, which is water-soluble. It has a bitter taste and may lead to taste disturbance. It also has the potential to cause tooth staining and to increase calculus formation. Chlorhexidine gluconate remains active in the mouth for a long time after use. It is added to mouthwash, but it is very difficult to formulate into toothpaste. Chlorhexidine acetate, which is less soluble than the gluconate, is used in some products, but not toothpaste.

Domiphen Bromide:

Domiphen bromide (known as "bradasol" in the brand Binaca) is a broad-spectrum antimicrobial similar to CPC. It is also used in conjunction with CPC to fight bad breath—as used in Scope mouthwash (Procter & Gamble). Domiphen bromide is difficult to formulate in a standard toothpaste.

Fluoride:

Fluoride may be included in oral health products in many forms, including:

- Sodium fluoride (NaF)
- Sodium monofluorophosphate (SMFP)
- "-amine" fluoride

Fluoride has several actions that are useful from the oral health perspective. It strengthens the teeth against caries by making the enamel less soluble and by promoting remineralization. At the same time, it may help with plaque acid control: fluoride interferes with the metabolism of plaque bacteria and so may help inhibit plaque acid production.

It has also been suggested that fluoride helps to treat sensitivity by promoting remineralization, which blocks the open tubules in dentin. However, neither the UK Department of Health (DoH) nor the US Federal Drug Authority (FDA) accepts this claim.

Gantrez (PVM/MA Co-polymer):

Gantrez is a copolymer of polyvinyl methyl ether (PVM) and maleic acid (MA). In combination with triclosan, it is a patented system that is used to improve the retention of triclosan in the mouth (Colgate Total). However, no published clinical study proves the ability of Gantrez to enhance the activity of triclosan. There *is* laboratory data supporting its effectiveness. Long-term clinical trials indicate that triclosan/Gantrez combinations are effective against plaque, gingivitis, calculus, and caries. This led to FDA approval of Colgate Total and was the first time the agency had cleared an active ingredient for the prevention of gingivitis, plaque, and cavities. Colgate Total was the first toothpaste to carry the American Dental Association seal for prevention of plaque, gingivitis, cavities, and calculus. Gantrez is also used in combination with pyrophosphate to improve effectiveness against calculus.

Glucose Oxidase (GOx) and Amyloglucosidase (AMG):

Glucose oxidase and amyloglucosidase are enzymes claimed to boost the levels of peroxide in saliva, which subsequently attacks plaque. These enzymes are included in some products indicated for the treatment of plaque and gingivitis. However, data supporting their effectiveness is inconclusive. They are used in Zendium (Oral-B) toothpaste.

Great Teeth for Life

Hexetidine ($C_{21}H_{45}N_3$):

Hexetidine is a broad-spectrum antimicrobial that is similar to chlorhexidine. It has moderate anti-plaque and antimicrobial activity but little effect in gingivitis compared with chlorhexidine. The antibacterial activity of hexetidine has been enhanced by combining it with metal ions such as zinc or copper. Hexetidine remains in the mouth for a reasonable length of time after use (for a shorter period than chlorhexidine but longer than CPC). As with the chlorhexidine salts, hexetidine has a bitter taste, may cause taste disturbance, is difficult to formulate as a toothpaste, and occasionally causes tooth staining. Stability can be a problem, and hexetidine is poorly soluble in water. It has no technical advantage over chlorhexidine.

Hydrogen Peroxide (H_2O_2):

Hydrogen peroxide is a bleaching agent with antimicrobial effects, and it has been used historically, at high concentrations, for the treatment of severe gingivitis. Adverse effects associated with hydrogen peroxide can include tissue injury, delayed wound healing, and a risk of overgrowth by *Candida albicans* if used regularly over a period of time. Weakening of the tooth enamel can occur with long-term use of hydrogen peroxide. Its use is permitted in the United States up to a level of 3 percent w/w, while in the EU it is limited to 0.1 percent w/w. In Canada, it is limited to short-period professional use only—up to fourteen days.

Natural Oils and Flavors:

The natural oils and flavors used in oral healthcare products—for example, Listerine—include wintergreen, eucalyptus oil, menthol, and thymol. It has been suggested that natural oils may work by reducing the levels of bacterial toxins in the plaque. A mixture of essential oils has been in use as mouthwash for over a century. These oils (thymol, eucalyptol, methyl salicylate, menthol) can reduce preformed plaque and inhibit further development of existing plaque and gingivitis. Long-term rinsing with essential oils has also been reported to reduce the levels of endotoxin in plaque, which could be of significance in preventing inflammation.

Papain:

Papain is a naturally occurring enzyme that dissolves protein. There is some evidence to show that the combination of papain and citrate can remove superficial tooth staining. Papain is used in Rembrandt toothpaste.

Potassium Nitrate (KNO_3):

Like strontium, potassium has a desensitizing effect. The exact mode of action of potassium nitrate has not yet been established. Initially, it was thought that potassium citrate desensitization of dentin following application of potassium nitrate resulted through closure of the dentin tubules by a process of crystal formation.

Other investigators, however, have suggested that potassium desensitization occurs because of raising the potassium concentration within the dentin tubules, rendering the nerves less sensitive to further stimuli by depolarizing the nerve membrane. Potassium nitrate is the active ingredient used in Aquafresh Sensitive in the United States. Potassium chloride and potassium citrate are used in some competitor products outside the United States.

Pyrophosphates:

Sodium and/or potassium pyrophosphates are included in oral health-care products as anti-tartar agents. They inhibit the formation of crystals and are therefore indicated for the prevention of calculus. However, the patent situation is very complicated and affects the freedom to formulate in this area. The salty taste of pyrophosphate is a problem that has to be overcome in the product formulation.

Sanguinarine:

Sanguarine is a natural plant extract reported to have in vitro broad-spectrum antimicrobial effects in the mouth. The supporting data are difficult to interpret since sanguinarine has been mainly used in combination with zinc, which has recognized effects of its own. There is evidence to show that sanguinarine prevents plaque bacteria from sticking to the teeth, which may be able to slow the conversion of sugar to plaque acid. The evidence is inconclusive, and as a result, sanguinarine has never received a product license in the United Kingdom.

Sodium Lauryl Sulphate (SLS) and Sodium Tripolyphosphate (STP):

SLS is a foaming, cleaning, and dispersing product. It is also an effective bactericidal agent in its own right. STP has an effect similar to that of pyrophosphate. It slows the growth of crystals, inhibiting the formation and growth of calculus. At higher concentrations, as in Aquafresh and Macleans whitening toothpastes, STP denatures (breaks down) the stain matrix. It does this by removing calcium bridges between the stain molecules and surface proteins on the teeth, making the stain easier to remove.

Stannous Fluoride (SnF_2):

Stannous fluoride generally has the same effects as fluoride. However, recent evidence from in vitro and human clinical studies indicates that stannous fluoride also has antibacterial properties, as well as the ability to reduce dentin hypersensitivity. These therapeutic benefits seem to be mainly attributable to the stannous ion (tin). There are drawbacks, however: there is a reasonable risk that stannous fluoride will stain the teeth, and it can be difficult to achieve a stable formulation of products based on stannous fluoride. Crest use stannous fluoride in its gum care toothpaste in the United States.

Strontium Acetate ($Sr(C_2H_3O_2)_2$) and Strontium Chloride ($SrCl_2$):

As discussed previously, agents based on strontium reduce the pain from sensitive teeth by blocking the tubules in the exposed dentin.

Triclosan ($C_{12}H_7Cl_3O_2$):

Triclosan is a broad-spectrum antibacterial agent used for the last twenty-five years in soaps, deodorants, cosmetics, and other dermatological preparations. A more recent indication for Triclosan is in preventative dentistry as an ingredient in toothpaste and mouthwash to increase the efficacy of bacterial plaque removal from teeth and to reduce gingivitis. There is some evidence that triclosan inhibits the formation of plaque on clean surfaces. At low concentrations, it interferes with the uptake of nutrients into bacterial cells and is bacteriostatic. At higher concentrations, triclosan is bactericidal, as it disrupts the plasma membrane, resulting in leakage of cellular components and cell death. It is also reported to have anti-inflammatory activity. Laboratory investigations indicate that triclosan can inhibit the formation of important mediators of inflammation. Triclosan is insoluble in water, although the organic solvent or oil used to solubilise Triclosan in mouthwash can influence its effectiveness.

Addition of a copolymer (Gantrez, as used in Colgate Total) has been shown to improve staying power in the mouth and increase efficacy. The combination of triclosan plus zinc citrate (as used by Unilever) has been shown to prevent gingivitis and reduce calculus formation.

Xylitol ($C_5H_{12}O_5$):

Xylitol is an artificial sweetener derived from silver birch trees. It does not appear to be metabolized by oral bacteria to form acid and indeed, in vitro, on entering the cell, xylitol is phosphorylated to form an inhibitory compound. Xylitol in chewing gum is reported to reduce the numbers of Streptococcus mutans in plaque and saliva, as well as reduce the amount of plaque present. The exact mode of action is not known, but it is claimed to cause intracellular accumulation of a particular form of phosphorylated xylitol, xylitol-5-phosphate, and a subsequent reduction in the ability of the bacteria to produce acid.

However, it has not been ascertained in vivo whether xylitol has the potential to reduce plaque quantity by altering metabolic traits of the bacteria. Indeed, recent work in young adults with a low incidence of caries suggests that exposure of the oral cavity to acceptable doses of xylitol has no effect on the microbial deposits on the teeth. The digestion of large amounts of xylitol can cause diarrhea.

Zinc Citrate ($C_{12}H_{10}O_{14}Zn_3$) (Zinc Chloride—$ZnCl_2$):

Zinc citrate is a metal salt that exerts an antimicrobial effect by inhibiting a variety of bacterial enzyme reactions, including the breakdown of sugar into plaque acid. There is evidence that the effect of zinc salts in reducing plaque enhances those of other antimicrobials. Interestingly, zinc salts seem to have a synergistic antibacterial effect when combined with drugs such as hexetidine, triclosan, and chlorhexidine. Zinc, used in combination with other substances, has been shown to reduce calculus. It should be noted, however, that zinc salts can bind to proteins, which may reduce their efficacy in the mouth. Zinc citrate (and zinc chloride) was originally used in Signal.

All these chemicals have very minor adverse reactions in either the mouths or the bodies of the users. Taking a global view, it must be conceded that billions of applications of toothpaste over many years have not led to health problems. On a personal note, the only toothpaste to make my gums ulcerate was one made from completely natural ingredients!

Which Toothpaste to Use?

Patients are always asking their dentists for recommendations, and often they will simply be given samples of what the dentist has been sent by the manufacturers. There is little difference between most of them.

Toothpaste must not be swallowed, especially when used by a child. Most children's toothpastes do have a much smaller percentage of fluoride for this reason.

Some toothpastes are more abrasive than others, and for this reason I cannot recommend the smoker's tooth powder for general use. Some of the larger manufacturers are introducing new toothpaste that becomes progressively less abrasive as you brush. It starts relatively abrasively to clean off the initial layers of plaque, but as you continue to brush, it becomes finer in order to give the teeth a good polish. The advantages would be twofold. The teeth would be much smoother after brushing, but also, knowing that this effect was taking place, people would tend to spend much longer on brushing their teeth, and that is desirable!

Colored or striped toothpastes are a bit of a gimmick, I believe, and most dentists would advise that white toothpaste should be used, so that when you spit out the foam and saliva, any blood from the gums can be easily seen.

For people with sensitive teeth, I recommend the desensitizing toothpastes, for they seem to work. Fluoride and strontium appear to be the active ingredients.

How much toothpaste should you use? Well, as little as possible is the simple answer. The manufacturers are to blame here, as they illustrate their wares in great profitable wedges on a brush. Not only is this unnecessary, wasteful, and perhaps hazardous, but it would foam up to an enormous degree and you wouldn't be able to see what you are doing. A tiny squeeze of paste is all that is necessary for babies, children, and adults alike.

Flossing

History

Dental floss is an ancient invention. Researchers have found dental floss and toothpick grooves in the teeth of prehistoric humans. Levi Spear Parmly (1790–1859), a New Orleans dentist, is credited as being the inventor of modern dental floss (or maybe the term reinventor would be more accurate). Parmly promoted teeth flossing with a piece of silk thread in 1815.[104]

In 1882, the Codman and Shurtleff Company of Randolph, Massachusetts, started to mass-produce unwaxed silk floss for commercial home use. The Johnson & Johnson Company of New Brunswick, New Jersey, was the first to patent dental floss in 1898. During WWII, Dr. Charles C. Bass developed nylon floss as a replacement for silk floss. Dr. Bass was also responsible for making teeth flossing an important part of dental hygiene.

Most dentists and hygienists agree that the standard advice for home care is brushing and flossing. Indeed, brushing is only half the cleaning story, as the floss is vital for getting into the spaces between the teeth, where even the most sensitive and sophisticated brush filaments cannot reach. In theory, with good brushing and good flossing, you could almost achieve 100 percent efficiency in cleaning. In practice, however, there are problems, and flossing can have its disadvantages. The major benefit of flossing, apart from its cleaning power, is that it familiarizes you with your own mouth. By flossing, you can become intimate with the geography of your mouth, with the number of teeth, with the spaces, with the nooks and crannies, with the places where food becomes trapped.

Once you start to use floss and do so regularly, your mouth and teeth will become part of your body, no longer a mere orifice and chewing instrument for food, and you can build up a special relationship. Fanciful perhaps, but infinitely valuable, and floss can encourage it.

How to Floss Your Teeth

Working in front of a mirror, take about forty-five to sixty centimeters (eighteen to twenty-four inches) of floss and wind each end around the middle finger of each hand, leaving about fifteen centimeters (six inches) between the fingers. Tighten the floss between thumb

---

104 (a) Dental Floss History. http://www.toothbrushexpress.com/html/floss_history.html
(b) http://en.wikipedia.org/wiki/Dental_floss#History

and forefinger. Gently guide the floss between two teeth until you touch the gum and feel a gentle pressure. The floss will look as though it's penetrating the gum, but it will be going into the crevice and disorganizing any plaque there. Pull the floss into a C-shape around the side of one tooth. Gently guide the floss down or up the tooth in a wiping motion, away from the gum, and then do the same with the other tooth. Wind on some fresh floss with your fingers, and repeat the procedure between every gap, on every tooth. Flossing does undoubtedly require a fair amount of manual dexterity, but with practice you will soon become more adept.

Types of Floss

Floss comes in waxed or unwaxed rolls, in precut lengths, or as a plastic tape, and it can be used in the hands or in special floss dispensers. A waxed tape, which is normally wider, could be useful for the first-time user or for children, as it runs between the teeth more easily, and there is less likelihood of fraying. It also tends to be more hygienic, as it doesn't get permeated with plaque. As the unwaxed floss is not coated, it will go between even finer gaps and will splay to cover a wider area. Flossers, which are becoming more popular, are an easier way of using floss.

The Disadvantages of Floss

Flossing can show up faulty dentistry. If there are ledges or overhangs on fillings or teeth, the floss will point them out. If the floss frays on these ledges or a rough edge of a crown, it can catch and be a source of irritation in itself. If floss is used wrongly, it can cut into the gums and cause damage. An incorrect backward and forward movement might even wear the tooth away at the gum line. If there is a large chunk of food caught between the teeth, floss can sometimes push the food farther into the gum. Again, an educational session with a hygienist or dental health educator will vastly improve your home care technique.

Disclosing Tablets

For cleaning the gaps between the teeth, there is now a vast array of oral hygiene aids. Remember, we are all individuals, so oral hygiene techniques will alter. Disclosing tablets should be used in conjunction with brushing and flossing as a way of finding plaque deposits. Disclosing tablets are composed of a vegetable dye, usually 4 percent erythrosine, and the flavoring agent. As with anything else to be used in the mouth, they should be, and probably are, nontoxic, nonallergenic, and nonirritating. They work on the principle that they stain the plaque layer blue or dark pink, and some are quite sophisticated in that they stain in different shades depending on the thickness of the plaque.

Especially with children, normally aged seven years or older (depending on the eruption of the permanent incisors), disclosing tablets should be used once a week to check plaque control. After the teeth have been brushed and flossed in the normal way then one tablet should be chewed, mixed with saliva, and gently swished around the teeth. The solution should then be spit out and the mouth rinsed with water. By looking in the mirror, the plaque will show as stained areas and should be brushed off thoroughly. It is a great way of learning the habit of efficient brushing.

Mouthwashes

The most natural, and sometimes the most effective, mouthwash is a solution of salty water, and this is particularly useful in reducing oral infections such as inflammation around an erupting wisdom tooth. To make this effective and low-cost mouthwash, add as much salt as will dissolve in a small tumbler full of hot or warm water. The water should be taken into the mouth and held over the inflammation for as long as possible, normally about one minute, before being spit out. The concentrated salt water draws out some of the pus and fluid from the tissues so that there is less inflammation. At such a high concentration, the salt solution will act as a local disinfectant. When used for mouth ulcers, though, it will make them sting! A big advantage of warm saltwater mouthwashes is that they are completely natural.

Proprietary mouthwashes can serve a useful purpose. Most are antiseptic and antibacterial and could unbalance the oral flora if used too frequently. Holistically, I would not recommend their use, except when advised by a dentist.

A disinfectant that is effective against gum disease is chlorhexidine, which can also be used at home. Chlorhexidine does undoubtedly work in a number of ways: by suppressing the oral bacteria, inhibiting plaque and calculus formation, and even dissolving plaque. On the debit side, however, the balance of the oral flora can be altered, it can cause staining on the teeth, it has an unpleasant taste, and it suppresses the taste buds.

Chlorhexidine also seems to help reduce the size and duration of mouth ulcers, although not their incidence. One should seek the advice of his or her dentist before using this chemical disinfectant.

Toothpicks and Wood Points

Toothpicks come in all shapes, sizes, and materials: the rich still use gold, the Chinese use ivory or plastic, the smart set use cocktail sticks, and the needy or desperate use the ends of matches! None will really do an efficient job of plaque removal because they will not curve to adapt to the contour of the tooth. They will be effective in fishing out the lumps of food. Proprietary wood points can be effective. As they are soft and usually sensibly shaped, areas of food trapping can be relieved, although they are not a great deal of use in plaque control. Using soft wood points minimizes the likelihood of damaging the gums by impaling them.

In Conclusion

These are the broad outlines of how you can help yourself at home by getting rid of plaque, the main causative factor of both tooth decay and gum disease. There are certain things, however, that only a dentist and her team can do.

Dental professionals, i.e., hygienists, therapists, and dental health educators, are now undertaking the role and responsibility of oral hygiene. This part of the dental team is specifically trained to provide an invaluable role in dental health prevention.

In modern dental practice, the emphasis is placed on the team approach in order to provide a professional, caring service to prevent dental disease.

CHAPTER NINE

Going to the Dentist: And You Thought It Was Just about Your Teeth!

Dentistry today is a specialist science, and every general dental practitioner is a highly skilled professional who has undergone a long and intensive training. The image of the dentist as a tooth puller has changed dramatically in a comparatively short time, and dentists have gone on the offensive. Their practices are now oriented towards prevention and restoration. Advances in research and material science have given dentists the weapons with which they can achieve these aims.

There has been controversy recently over how often one should visit the dentist. I unequivocally recommend the six-month interval as the ideal. The significance of those six months is perhaps arbitrary, but in practice, within that timescale, the progress of disease can be monitored and checked. It is unlikely that we would see new cavities occurring at such frequent intervals, but preventative measures could be introduced to arrest any areas where there are signs of early tooth decay. Gum disease, which can develop much more rapidly, often requires an even more frequent professional appraisal. Most of my patients see the hygienist every six months as a minimum. This time interval is often shortened if the severity of the patient's gum disease is increasing due to poor oral hygiene, lifestyle stresses, poor nutrition, etc.

Because the mouth is a barometer of health, regular inspection may reveal early signs of systemic disease. Mouth cancer is on the increase throughout the westernized world. Regular attendance and early detection can literally be the difference between life and death!

Dental Examinations

During their long training, dentists study many aspects of general medicine that are necessary to dental practice. Seemingly irrelevant medical information may have a profound influence on how the dentist interprets dental problems, and it will influence the treatment thereafter. Thus every dentist is, in a sense, holistic, in that he will be considering more than just the mouth, especially when undertaking the initial examination.

The Medical History

When you visit a dentist for the first time, you are confronted with a barrage of questions, including a written questionnaire. Many of these questions involve your past medical history, and although they could occasionally seem to be a little too private coming from a person who's supposed to be only concerned with filling your teeth, these questions are asked for specific reasons. It may seem particularly impertinent, for example, when a dentist asks a single female patient if she is on the contraceptive pill; however, as we have already seen, this may be relevant if there are any gum problems.

If the dentist asks whether you have had rheumatic fever as a child, it is because there is a unique, potentially fatal relationship between the consequences of the disease and some dental treatment.

Rheumatic fever, which a doctor would normally diagnose, occurs most commonly in childhood. It can start with a sore throat, make the joints and limbs painful and swollen, and the kidneys can also be affected. It's unlikely that you would be unaware of having this disease, as it can cause considerable distress for as long as eight to twelve weeks, the person being bed bound and ill.

A major consequence of rheumatic fever is that it may damage the lining and valves of the heart. Should certain bacteria that live in the mouth escape into the bloodstream and gain access to these areas of damaged tissue in the heart, a very serious infection can occur—SBE (subacute bacterial endocarditis).

If untreated, this can lead to heart failure and death. Dental treatment given routinely, such as a scaling or a dental extraction, can give rise to this bacterial release into the bloodstream. People who have a history of rheumatic fever may also have a heart murmur, although this is not always the case. It is vital for anyone who has had rheumatic fever to maintain scrupulous oral hygiene, and it is vital that he inform his dentist.

The same principles apply to any person who has had heart surgery, especially that involving valve replacement, and also to major prosthetic surgery such as hip replacements. Given this knowledge, the dentist can make the necessary safeguards. The usual precautions consist of giving the patient an appropriate antibiotic prior to the dental treatment. The dentist may consult with the patient's medical consultant if there is any doubt relating to the correct treatment protocol.

Questions about your liver or whether you have ever been jaundiced are relevant to transmittable viral diseases such as hepatitis. Hepatitis A is highly contagious via the blood, and although fully recovered, the sufferer may still be a carrier of the virus for many years afterwards. The dentist will need to know this so that he can take all the appropriate safeguards.

The barrage may continue with questions on whether you are taking any medications or drugs, whether you smoke, drink to excess, have any allergies, have had any major operations or neurological symptoms, and so on. In fact, virtually everything that a doctor would need to know for a thorough insurance medical.

Dentists may also ask whether you suffer from migraines or frequent headaches or from chronic pain in your back and/or other parts of the body. A dentist will find significance in the answers you give, for they may relate to a jaw condition known as TMJ (temporomandibular joint) syndrome (see page 181). At this stage, the questions may even elicit information about past involvement in car accidents, etc., and any other osteopathic stresses that you might have suffered.

The above are just a few examples of medical conditions that have a real relevance to your dental condition and subsequent treatment.

The Dental History

After the medical questions, the dental questions will be asked. The primary question is usually something to the effect of, "Are you experiencing any pain or problems with your teeth or gums?" Another priority question should be, "Do your gums bleed?" We all now know the ramifications of that! For new patients, it is relevant for the dentist to know the last time you had any treatment, as this will indicate the rate of progress of any dental disease, especially the accumulation of dental plaque and calculus. If there is any pain or discomfort, the dentist will want you to be specific about its nature, location, type, intensity, frequency, and duration, as well as what stimulus brings on the pain. From this verbal interrogation alone, much can be gleaned about the condition of the teeth and gums.

The holistic dentist will also be interested to know about clicking and creaking noises on opening and closing the jaws. In addition, he will want to know if you grind your teeth, have frequent sinusitis, dizziness, ringing or popping in the ears, or if you experience a feeling that your teeth don't meet properly. If the answers to any of the above are affirmative, this could indicate a jaw dysfunction. Questions that might also have a nutritional significance may be asked, such as whether you have frequent ulcers, a sore tongue, cold sores, bad breath, or a dry mouth. Depression, and the drugs used to treat it, can cause a dry mouth due to a reduction of the flow of saliva. Patients with a dry mouth, from any medical condition, have a greater likelihood of developing tooth decay and gum disease.

Physical Impressions

First impressions count. Those initial summings-up are often subconscious, but the holistic dentist will deliberately include them as part of the examination and may well make copious notes to that effect. How many people notice, and realize the significance of, a crooked smile, a nose that slopes to one side of the face, or one eye that does not open as much as the other? How many people are conscious of one shoulder lower than the other (likewise with the breasts), one leg longer than the other, or an incorrectly postured head? The holistic dentist regards all these seemingly minor aberrations with professional interest, for once again they could be signs of skeletal imbalance that in turn may affect the correct functioning of the jaw.

As soon as you sit in the dental chair, the dentist will be able to observe the color of your complexion, the texture of your hair and skin, the condition of your eyes, any rashes or spots, or irregular swellings on either the face or neck. Ruddy cheeks could suggest high blood pressure. Lifeless hair could mean a recent illness or being below par; a hairdresser would come to the same conclusion. Protruding eyes may indicate an overactive thyroid. Rashes or spots could indicate hormonal imbalances, allergies, or mineral and vitamin deficiencies. Nails could show circulatory problems or deficiencies such as certain types of anemia or a deficiency of zinc (white spots). These are simply indications, and neither dentist, nor doctor for that matter, would immediately rush to a firm diagnosis. A practitioner, like a detective, is building a health picture of his patient.

Before looking in your mouth, the dentist may want to feel your neck and jaw muscles to see if there are any irregularities, swollen glands, or inflammation in the tissues surrounding the mouth. Do not be alarmed if the dentist sticks a finger in either ear or shouts at you to open and close your mouth! He will be investigating the way in which the jaw mechanisms are working.

Open Wide, Please

The big moment has arrived. The dentist will look into your mouth, which is what you thought he would have done right at the beginning. Before actually examining the teeth, the dentist will have a good look around at all parts of the mouth: the lips, cheek tissue, palate, tongue, floor of the mouth, and as far back as the tonsils. Many of these areas have a clinical significance.

The tongue has always been used as an indicator of health. Think of the doctor asking you to stick your tongue out. A number of medical conditions can reveal themselves; for example, a vitamin B deficiency can make the tongue a deeper red in color, giving a raw steak appearance. Heavy smoking or medical drug taking can give rise to a discolored or a "hairy" tongue, which can look alarming, as the back of the tongue literally has long strands growing from it, and these can grow so long that they break off!

Your dentist will be looking for any unusual lumps such as blocked salivary ducts, mumps, enlarged lymph nodes, or even a chronic abscess from a tooth. Also, the dental examination (checkup) is an opportunity for your dentist to perform a health screen for mouth cancer.

A common condition often confused with early signs of mouth cancer is lichen planus. This condition is not a form of cancer. Lichen planus often manifests as white streaks on the cheek tissue, but it may also be seen on other parts of the mouth, including the gums, the tongue, palate, and lips. Most experts agree that lichen planus is a response to stress and occurs most frequently in middle-aged adults. I believe this disease is a result of modern-day lifestyle stresses, including deficient nutrition.

An experienced practitioner can glean an enormous amount of information from this initial study of the mouth, not least from the texture, color, and overall appearance of the tissues. The interior of the mouth is hardy and resilient, and it does not readily succumb to infection or damage. This is borne out by the fact that the majority of the population has little sign of disease in the soft tissues of the mouth.

On examining the gums, even the mildest inflammation will be immediately apparent to the dentist. High on the priority list is to care for the foundation of the teeth, that is, the gums and the jaw structure supporting the teeth. The dentist will examine the gums carefully and, if there are any problems, will discuss these with the patient. By explaining the situation to the patient, an effective action plan can be implemented. Most of the preventative treatment is carried out at home, so patient motivation is crucial. Normally the hygienist will implement any treatment that is necessary at the dental practice.

Oddly enough, the teeth are examined last of all. Dentists will be looking for dental cavities, at the condition of existing fillings and crowns, and at the relationship between the individual teeth. They will also look for signs of excessive wear, perhaps due to overenthusiastic brushing; abrasion on the biting surfaces, which may indicate grinding; and at how the top and bottom teeth come together. Erosion, or the chemical wearing away of the teeth, possibly caused by too high a citrus fruit and acidic drink intake, can be spotted at this stage as well. Due to the increase in the consumption of fizzy and carbonated drinks, many of our children are suffering from thinning and sensitive teeth, a manifestation of teeth erosion.

By virtue of the intense light, the dentist can easily see many of the above and because the teeth are, to a certain extent, translucent, can often detect the earliest signs of tooth decay, which may not be picked up by a dental probe. To increase their detective powers, many dentists use magnification.

The relationship between the teeth and gums is what the dentist is primarily interested in because therein lies the origins of dental disease. As previously discussed, the shape, position, the crowding, and the function are all contributory factors, and at this time the dentist will be able to assess the effect these may have singularly on the condition of the patient's dental health. Poor hygiene will reveal itself now. It is often a source of amusement for many dentists when a child presents for examination with red and sore gums due to the unaccustomed extra brushing effort immediately beforehand. The presence of a large buildup of calculus and plaque will reveal the areas of the mouth that are habitually brushed less efficiently.

Based on all these findings, the dentist will have a clear picture not just of the mouth, but also of the general health and well-being of the patient. Further investigations may be required if the dentist feels they are necessary. He may take X-rays, take models of the teeth, refer the patient on to a dental specialist, recommend nutritional counseling or attendance with an osteopath, or he may wish to liaise with the patient's general medical practitioner.

Mouth Cancer

I have deliberately left this increasingly common but nasty disease until now. As a dental-medical priority, screening for mouth cancer is top of the list, an opportunity for a dentist to save lives by early detection.

Globally, more than four hundred thousand new cases are reported each year. In Europe, around a hundred thousand people are diagnosed with head and neck cancers, with about forty thousand dying from these diseases. In the United States, nearly thirty thousand develop mouth cancer every year, with one person dying every hour of every day. Men are twice as likely to be affected as women, particularly men over forty years old.[105]

Cancer can occur in any part of the mouth, tongue, lips, throat, salivary glands—in fact, any part of the head and neck. Mouth cancers have a greater likelihood of death compared to breast cancer, cervical cancer, or skin melanomas.

In the early stages, mouth cancer can be difficult to detect and can be painless. The British Dental Health Foundation (BDHF)—www.dentalhealth.org.uk—gives excellent advice on oral health issues. Here are their guidelines concerning mouth cancer:

---

105 (a) "Mouth Cancer Awareness, Oral Cancer in Throat, Tongue, Jaw, Head and Neck," Mouth Cancer Foundation. http://www.rdoc.org.uk/
(b) "Mouth Cancer," British Dental Health Foundation. http://www.dentalhealth.org.uk/faqs/
(c) The Oral Cancer Foundation, May 5. 2009 http://oralcancerfoundation.org/

Brian Halvorsen, BDS, LDS RCS

Early Detection of Mouth Cancer Is Vital

Mouth cancer kills one person every five hours in the United Kingdom, and the number of new cases is increasing every year.

Smoking is the most common cause of the condition. It turns saliva into a deadly cocktail that damages cells in the mouth and can turn them cancerous. Smoking increases a person's risk of developing mouth cancer by around five times.

Other forms of smokeless tobacco such as chewing tobacco, paan, areca nut, and gutkha are similarly dangerous and are all habits favored by some ethnic groups.

Excessive consumption of alcohol is also a major risk factor. The type of alcohol consumed does not affect a person's mouth cancer risk. Beer, wine, and spirits are equally damaging.

It is recommended that men drink no more than three to four units per day and women no more than two to three. A unit is the equivalent of a glass of wine, a single measure of spirits, or a half pint of beer, lager, or cider.

It should be noted that, with regard to mouth cancer, the effects of the two habits actually multiply together, and people who use both tobacco and alcohol to excess are up to a staggering thirty times more likely to develop the condition.

A poor diet can also be a contributory factor for mouth cancer, and it is recommended that people eat a healthy, balanced diet, including at least five portions of fruit and vegetables each day, while cutting down on the consumption of fat, salt, and sugar.

Early detection and treatment of mouth cancer increases a person's survival chances, from only one in two, to around nine out of ten. So it is important that people are aware of common early symptoms.

Early signs of mouth cancer can include a non-healing mouth ulcer, a lump, or a red or white patch in the mouth.

However, mouth cancer can strike in a number of different places, including the lips, the tongue, and the gums and cheek, so it is important that people examine their own mouths on a regular basis.

Less common early symptoms can include pain on chewing or swallowing, a sore throat that won't go away, and unusual pain, bleeding, or numbness in the cheek.

As these could easily be mistaken for something less serious, it is recommended that people maintain regular visits to the dentist. People should book additional appointments if they have any concerns.

I cannot stress how important it is to visit the dentist every six months. This has become a controversial issue, as some authorities are saying a yearly checkup or even longer is sufficient. From the above, you can see that even if your teeth and gums are in reasonable order, a regular oral health screen will not only catch any disease in its early stages, but will also give you reassurance that all is okay.

Nutrition plays a pivotal role in preventative dentistry, especially concerning mouth cancer. However, if we define nutrition as any intake the body experiences, smoking and excessive consumption of alcohol are of disease-causing *mal*nutrition.

CHAPTER TEN

Stress, Stress, Stress, Stress—Four Reasons Why You Are Ill

In any conversation, it doesn't take long before the subject of health crops up, and in fact, this is the very first greeting most people receive: "How are you?" Very often this can lead into a blow-by-blow account of the latest malady, be it major or minor. If a visitor from outer space were to examine the vast majority of people on the planet, he would have to conclude that we were a nation of health cripples. In fact, one commentator has suggested that "we are standing on the very edge of the abyss of a crisis of epidemic magnitude, such as the world has never known before, including chronic poisoning, heart and artery disease, cerebral strokes, diseases of the nervous system, mental and emotional disorders, rampant dental decay, congenital malformations, and degenerative conditions of all sorts" (Nutrition Science and Health Education, Dr. C. Curtis Shears).[106]

If you don't believe me, then how does 175 million working days lost with certified illness sound? This is in England alone! Costing the country in excess of £100 billion ($162 billion), and all in one year! When you examine the waiting lists for major surgical operations, all as a result of some form of disease, the numbers are staggering—*one in twenty* of the entire population. Is the cost of

---

106 (a) "Ill Health Costs Economy £100bn." BBC News, March 17, 2008. http://news.bbc.co.uk/1/hi/health/7297174.stm
(b) "The Burden of Food Related Ill Health in the UK, Bio-Medicine," *BMJ Specialty Journals*, November 14, 2005. http://news.bio-medicine.org/medicine-news-3/The-burden-of-foodrelated-ill-health-in-the-UK-7659-1/
(c) Reinhardt, U. "Why Does U.S. Health Care Cost So Much?" *The New York Times*, November 14, 2008. http://economix.blogs.nytimes.com/2008/11/14/why-does-us-healthcare-cost-so-much-part-i/

the National Health Service diminishing? The answer is a categorical no, and we are still short of medical staff, equipment, and facilities. The future looks rather bleak. The majority of health-care systems throughout the world are based on cure rather than prevention. It's the ambulance at the base of the cliff, not the fence at the top.

Can we as individuals change this situation? I sincerely believe we can. Holistically we must take responsibility for our own welfare and that of our family. Good health is one of the most precious gifts humanity can strive for and maintain.

Stresses That Cause Disease

Many medical scientists and practitioners of all disciplines, including psychologists and philosophers, believe that the cause of the majority of diseases is multifactorial and primarily linked to our so-called "civilized society." This lifestyle is inextricably linked with stress. Many healers will often break this stress down into a number of categories, although all are interdependent. The major stresses may be defined in four broad categories: environmental, psychological, physical, and nutritional, not necessarily in that order of importance.

It is said that a certain amount of stress is good for us. Perhaps, as it may act as a form of motivation. But the level of stress is what is important, as too much will lead to ill health. Although in most westernized countries life expectancy is increasing, I believe that the quality of life is deteriorating. In the United States, more than five million people have Alzheimer's, and this is forecast to rise to sixteen million by 2050.[107] No wonder people worry about getting old! This, I believe, is an example of a condition that is age related, but it could be minimized if lifelong stresses were reduced.

Environmental

This is the one over which the average person has no individual control, although environmental groups are beginning to make

---

107 Alzheimer's Disease, Fisher Center for Alzheimer's Research, April 13, 2009 http://www.alzinfo.org/

their voices heard. It is not only the eccentrics in their smocks and sandals who are demanding change, but well-respected scientists, physicians, and many well-educated people, including politicians from all walks of life and from all over the world. What we as a society are doing to our global environment has already directly affected individual health. Think of the mercury being spewed out into the atmosphere by the Chinese fossil-burning power stations. Mercury, according to the World Health Organization, is the most environmentally toxic element on this planet. Environmentally, it makes Chernobyl seem like a bonfire in your garden!

It is universally agreed that if many of the directives shown below were followed, our environment would be dramatically improved.

1. Reduce industrial effluents. Look how the aquatic life in the Thames has proliferated since antipollution measures were taken. Think about how the smog of London was caused by the unchecked churning out of fumes from factory chimneys! How the Norwegians are protesting about the acid rain polluting their forests and rivers, a rain that is thought to originate in the United Kingdom! Every country on this planet has similar examples of successes and failures of their environmental care.

2. Phase out long-acting chemical pesticides and herbicides. Science should be used to develop natural and organic alternatives, which are biodegradable. By the use of chemicals such as DDT, whole populations of birds of prey were annihilated. What effect might these residues have on our bodies?

3. Recycle industrial and domestic wastes. This has obvious advantages in that it will not drain the earth of further valuable resources, and this is, to a limited extent, already carried out with glass and paper. The composting of food waste will return valuable trace elements to the soil.

4. Reduce the use of gasoline chemicals. A lot is known about the deleterious effects of car exhaust fumes, but much less is known about the harm that could be caused by chemical products in

food, water, air, pesticides, cosmetics, detergents, and drugs. When plastics dissolve or decompose, they release estrogenic esters responsible for hormonal problems for all forms of life, from fish to mankind.

The above are just a small sample of the environmental stresses that we face in the twenty-first century. I have not even mentioned global warming and its impact on our stress levels!

By cleaning up our environment, we will be improving the two most important nutrients mankind needs to survive: air and water. Being close to nature has proven health benefits. Even if you live in an apartment in the middle of a city, surround yourself with living plants and flowers, as they soak up negative energy. Improve your environment by utilizing colors, textures, shapes, and materials that create a sense of well-being and consequently reduce negative stressors. The ancient art of feng shui has helped many people reduce stress levels at their home and work environments.

Psychological

Negative emotional and spiritual stress has been shown[108] to chemically damage brain cells and make the individual more susceptible to diseases such as Alzheimer's.

It is well known, both in and outside of the medical profession, that the state of the mind plays a major role in the general health and well-being of the body. After the death of a loved one, it is not uncommon for the surviving partner to die within a fairly short space of time or to develop a serious illness of some sort, especially if the bond between them has been strong. Conversely, a patient who has been pronounced incurable can often have a remission entirely through determination and strength of will.

---

108 (a) Sawchenko, P. "Emotional Stress Could Be A Factor in Causing Alzheimer's," Salk Institute for Biological Studies, May 5, 2009. http://www.bio-medicine.org/medicine-news/Emotional-Stress-Could-Be-a-Factor-in-Causing-Alzheimers-3A-Study-20541-1/
(b) "The Human Brain— Stress." The Franklin Institute, Resources for Science Learning, 2004. http://www.fi.edu/learn/brain/stress.html

These are vivid illustrations, but we all suffer from less significant, but nonetheless important, day-to-day emotional stresses. Executives may regard their jobs as the most stressful but worry over how to manage the housekeeping or about an examination can create similar levels of stress in other individuals. We all react to stress in different ways, and every situation will elicit varying responses from differing individuals.

However, psychiatrists and researchers have drawn up a scale to help them measure life stress and find out how much stress piles up before illness sets in. "The Social Adjustment Rating Scale" (as taken from an article in the *Journal of Psychosomatic Research* by T. H. Holmes and R. H. Rahe[109]) is a list of forty-three stressful life events that can contribute to illness.

Reproduced here are the top fifteen, together with their grades:

Life Event:

1. Death of spouse (100)
2. Divorce (73)
3. Marital separation from spouse (65)
4. Detention in jail or other institution (63)
5. Death of a close family member (63)
6. Major personal injury or illness (53)
7. Marriage (50)
8. Being fired at work (47)
9. Marital reconciliation with mate (45)
10. Retirement from work (45)
11. Major change in the health or behavior of a family member (44)
12. Pregnancy (40)
13. Sexual difficulties (39)
14. Gaining a new family member (through birth, adoption, relative moving in) (39)
15. Major business readjustment (merger, reorganization, bankruptcy, etc.) (39)

---

109 Holmes and Rahe Stress Scale: http://en.wikipedia.org/wiki/Holmes_and_Rahe_stress_scale

In the twenty-first century, new surveys have shown[110] that as society becomes more affluent, people are often less happy and content. In fact, the opposite is true. Psychiatrists are using the term "Affluenza." The media—that is, television, radio, and newspapers—provides a form of pollution. We are constantly bombarded with politics and bad and depressing news and marketing messages that often have the overall effect of deflating our sense of well-being, leading to negativity and depression. Over the last thirty years, an antidote to all this doom and gloom has emerged: the lifestyle coaches. Some of my personal favorites are Deepak Chopra, Wayne Dyer, and John Gray (see bibliography). I believe that any religion or spiritual belief based on love, peace, wisdom, and reconciliation has an important role to play in reducing stress for individuals as well as in our societies.

Meditation is a superb way to reduce the stress of modern living. Once trained in a form of meditation, you can use your personal technique at home or work, on the train or plane—or in any situation where there is a moment of solitude. My own particular mantra is "'AHAH," which translates to *abundance, health, and happiness*.

I wish all my readers AHAH!

Physical

Any form of exercise will have health benefits: "Activity is life; stagnation is death."[111] Besides toning muscles, exercise improves the nervous system (used in recovery programs for victims of brain damage), the digestive system, the body metabolism, the circulatory system (especially the heart), the skeletal structure and associated muscles, the immune system, and the brain. Regular,

---

110 http://www.newessay.com/database/Afluenza-15837.html - Book Report on Afluenza

111 (a) http://health20-20.org/article.php?id=117 – Life is Activity, Stagnation is Death, Raymond O. West, MD, MPH
(b) http://www.hindustanlink.com/doctortex/doctor/exercising_to_keep_fit.htm - Exercising To Keep Fit

correct exercise benefits every vital organ of the body, as well as every biological function concerned with the process of living. In our toxic environment, exercise improves the excretion of toxins via sweat, urine, and feces.

There is a greater awareness these days of the need to keep in shape, and there has been an unprecedented boom in gymnasia, slimming clinics and health farms, and in participant sports, especially those requiring a lot of physical activity. Many more now believe in the old adage 'Mens sana in corpore sana,' which means 'A healthy mind in a healthy body.'

In times of danger, our ancestors produced hormones (adrenalins/ noradrenalins)[112] in their bodies, which better prepared them to either stand and fight or turn and flee. These hormones speeded up the heartbeat, increased blood pressure, tensed the muscles, and quickened the breathing. This was all very useful when facing that sabre-toothed tiger, but not so relevant when worrying about how to pay the gas bill—and today's stresses call forth the same hormones. If these induced hormones are not metabolized, they are inclined to build up and cause internal biochemical stress. This leads to depression, fatigue, mood swings, irritability, etc. Physical exercise is one of the best ways of reducing tension, and competitive sports are useful in releasing the chemical stressors by converting them into physical and mental aggression.

Posture, or the lack of it, can also contribute to physical stress on the body. If we sit, stand, or lie incorrectly, the bone structure and associated muscles are not in balance. These imbalances can lead to pain, discomfort, and degeneration. Many new sciences—like osteopathy, chiropractic, physiotherapy, and kinesiology—are evolving to combat and treat diseases that derive from these postural stresses.

---

112 (a) Fight or Flight Response: http://en.wikipedia.org/wiki/Fight-or-flight
(b) Neimark, N. "The Mind/Body Education Center, The Fight or Flight Response." http://www.thebodysoulconnection.com/Education Center/fight.html

Nutritional

We are what we ingest, and if you think about it, we can be nothing else. After all, what else are we made of but what we consume and what we breathe? If we feed ourselves with rubbish, the result is obvious.

In an ever-toxic environment, changing one's diet is possibly the easiest way of reducing physical stress. As this is the recurrent theme of this book, I will detail diet and supplementation as a separate section. Nutritional science can help prevent virtually all the common illnesses that befall us, including most cancers, neurodegenerative diseases such as clinical depression and dementias, heart and circulatory disease; in fact, the list is virtually endless. Nutrition is about prevention. This is why the earlier good dietary habits are introduced, the less likely preventable diseases will occur. Again, Dr. Price's observations in the 1930s illustrate in an unforgettable way the physical degeneration that occurs when human groups abandon nourishing traditional diets in favor of modern convenience foods.

The body digests food through a long and complicated process, which begins, as we know, in the mouth. If that food is of poor quality, overrefined, contaminated, laden with additives, and is in incorrect proportions for the body's requirements, there can be internal stresses. The entire digestive and metabolic system has to work harder to properly process the nutrients that the body requires.

It is often assumed that in the more developed countries, we do not suffer from malnutrition. However, vitamin and mineral deficiencies and their related diseases are becoming increasingly commonplace, and these, surprisingly, are often caused by overeating rather than by undereating. The overconsumption of empty calories found in refined sugar and carbohydrates, as well as the overconsumption of protein and fat, gives rise to the majority of the illnesses that fill our hospitals and dental chairs.

Perhaps we ought to take the advice of the "father of medicine," for Hippocrates wrote in 460 BC: "Foods must be in the condition in which they are found in nature, or at least in a condition as close as possible to that found in nature. Let your food be your medicine and your medicine your food."[113]

Stress and Disease

Many health professionals subscribe to the concept that if a person exceeds a certain stress threshold, then disease will result. Imagine a stress threshold of one hundred. If we give points for the above-mentioned stresses, which all have a cumulative effect on one's health or lack of it, then the higher the figure, the nearer to disease we come and vice versa. Let's take an example:

Mr. X has a poor diet due to eating on the run and snack foods. This will count for, say, thirty-five points; he lives in the center of the city, which adds on another thirty points. His job is sedentary, but he exercises twice a week, which adds fifteen points; and he has a happy marriage and a steady job, which means another ten. His total count is below the theoretical disease level, but if he moves to a new residence, a well-known stress factor, say, of twenty, Mr. X could complain of depression, headaches, back pain, and indigestion.

By lowering any or all of the contributory stresses, his health could be restored, although some aspects would be difficult to alter. Diet, however, can be simple to modify, and can often bring beneficial results in a short space of time. The ideal situation, therefore, is obviously one in which the levels of stress attached to each area of life are low, and we should all strive to this end.

Dentists may observe when their patients are suffering from levels of stress that may be affecting their immune system. Dentists are in a unique position to notice any health changes, as they will often be examining patients at regular intervals.

Verbally asking a patient how she is will often bring forth a response indicating the origins of her stress. An examination of the mouth

---

113 Clement, B. "The Hippocrates Health Institute: Healing Disease Through Living Foods." http://www.consumerhealth.org/articles/display.cfm?ID=19990303134731

may show the manifestations of the stress; this can be increases in gum disease, excessive wear on the teeth due to night grinding, and patients complaining of such things as dryness in the mouth and bad breath.

By further questioning and more detailed examination, perhaps including symptoms of the whole body, disease in its early stages may be diagnosed and, where necessary, referred to the patient's medical practitioner or another appropriate healer. The dentist could now be taking a new role in society by acting as an early-warning health screen, becoming involved in more direct health care such as nutritional counseling.

As a reminder, the word *holistic* means, in general terms, an involvement with the whole person. Many dentists, however, are reticent about considering treating any other parts of the body except the head and neck. Their training has concentrated on the anatomy, physiology, biochemistry, and disease of everything above the shoulders, and correctly so.

After all, they wanted to be specialists in the mouth. But it is becoming increasingly apparent that dentists will have to look beyond those boundaries if they want to play a greater role in the holistic treatment of their patients.

Dentistry and physical stress

TMJ Syndrome

A substantial proportion of the population suffers from migraines or frequent headaches. Over a third of these may have their origins in imbalance and malfunction of the joint that connects the lower jaw to the skull. This is called the temporomandibular joint (TMJ). Dysfunction of the TMJ can lead to a host of seemingly unrelated health problems. Although TMJ syndrome has been recognized for many years, it is only recently that the far-reaching bodily consequences have been appreciated. This is a classic example of where a holistic approach will pay handsome dividends in the understanding and treating of this common condition.

Many headaches, migraines, back and neck pains, dizzy spells, and ailments like chronic sinusitis, sore throats, tension, and insomnia can be the direct result of TMJ syndrome. Many osteopaths, for instance, have recognized that much back pain stems from a jaw dysfunction, and until recently, there has been little clinical exchange between them and the dental profession. Many TMJ syndrome sufferers are taking painkillers, muscle relaxants, and antidepressants because their symptoms have not been properly diagnosed or effectively treated.

The head weighs generally between nine to fourteen pounds (four to six kilograms) and balances on the end of a flexible pole, the spine. The muscles of the shoulders, neck, and lower jaw maintain that balance. When the latter is not balanced properly, the head can become misaligned and the supporting muscles will have to strain to keep it in its proper position on the neck. This can result in muscle strain and asymmetries throughout the whole body, not just the face and neck. Dentists would be looking out for any indication of this during the first visual and physical examination of their patients.

If TMJ syndrome is thought to be involved, muscles located as far apart as the temple and the calf of the leg may be palpated for signs of strain and tenderness. Don't suspect your dentist of less than professional motives; he is in pursuit of a clear diagnosis. X-rays of the jaw joints are also valuable, not only for establishing the way in which the lower jaw slots into its allotted place, but also to look for arthritis of the joint. The dentist, by placing his fingers in your ears, can also assess the position of the joints! Try it for yourself. Place a finger in your ear, press inwards and forwards, then open and close your mouth slowly. If you can feel the movement in the joint, if it is not the same on both sides, or if there is clicking, then there may be a potential Jaw dysfunction.

If there is a strong indication that TMJ syndrome is involved, then the dentist will take models of your teeth. These will provide valuable information about how your teeth interrelate, and will also provide the basis for making an appliance, which, it is hoped, will relieve the symptoms. In the majority of cases, by simply fitting a plastic cover to the top or bottom teeth, relief can be obtained. The appliance, often referred to as a "stress breaker" or "bite splint" appears to work by keeping the jaws in a nonhabitual position, giving the muscles time to relax and rearrange themselves from their previously stressed position. The appliance will need to be worn continuously, especially during periods of uninterrupted concentration, such as driving a car or writing a book, and particularly during sleep. Reduction of symptoms such as headaches, clicking jaws, back pain, and tinnitus (buzzing in the ears) can be noticed within a week or two. Once the symptoms have disappeared, the appliance should be retained for when stressful situations may build up in the future.

There are some sufferers who, to obtain relief, require a much more accurate method of determining the correct relationship between their jaws. The types of appliance they require have to be carefully measured and constructed, and may initially feel completely alien, as if wearing a brick in the mouth. There is usually rapid acceptance, especially when their symptoms and pain, as if by magic, completely disappear. Other health professionals may need to be brought in at this stage, including osteopaths, chiropractors, neurologists, doctors, and physiotherapists, who would, along with the dentist, provide a team approach in helping the patient.

Many people with lopsided or malfunctioning jaw joints do not suffer any symptoms, but they are walking time bombs in a sense. It is generally agreed that TMJ syndrome is brought on by stress, whether dietary, emotional, environmental, or physical, and if these stresses accumulate, they can trigger the vast range of TMJ-related complaints. To both new sufferers and all those who have experienced long-term pain, the knowledge and expertise of the dentist may offer hope.

CHAPTER ELEVEN

The Importance of Good Nutrition: Feed Your Mouth, Feed Your Body

Every person is genetically unique. The expression "One man's meat is another man's poison" is true. Generalized dietary advice, no matter how sound the principles, may not be compatible with a particular individual. I feel nutritional counseling should only be undertaken on a one-to-one basis, as it is essential to establish the individual nutritional status of the patient.

Following an extensive written and oral questioning of the client's medical and dietary history, most nutritionists can begin their counseling. I find that a blood test provides a scientific and accurate way of assessing the patient's nutritional status. By looking at the blood chemistry, the blood cells and the circulating levels of minerals and vitamins can be measured. The blood chemistry will tell us the existing condition of many of the vital organs and glands through the levels of chemicals like cholesterol, thyroid hormones, and albumin, etc. There are many, and they all have individual and combined significance. The condition and number of the blood cells is obviously important, especially concerning things such as anemia and chronic infections, but the level of certain minerals and vitamins is what is relevant to nutritional counseling. Any worrying abnormal results can be referred to the patient's medical practitioner.

The blood is not the only method, though; analysis of hair, sweat, urine, and feces can be of great value in giving a complete nutritional picture. If properly undertaken, hair analysis has the unique advantage of being able to show the effects of nutrition over several months of hair growth. There are analytical laboratories in most countries. Your nutritionist will know where to send the relevant tests for analysis.

If two people eat exactly the same food in the same quantities, the amount of nutrients that each person will absorb and metabolize from this food will differ. The blood analysis or other tests will indicate what is happening in the body, but the nutritionist will also want to know what food is being ingested to give these results. A diet sheet is one of the best ways of getting this information. The patient fills it in, listing everything he has eaten and drunk in a week (a shorter time wouldn't be appropriate). It is also important that the patient eats what he would normally consume during that week: a sudden guilty reliance on salads will not impress, and it will not lead to any accurate conclusions.

Shown below is an example of a diet sheet that can be filled in to provide evidence for what patients/clients have eaten on a daily basis.

Diet Sheet (include quantities/weights)

Breakfast	Lunch	Dinner	Additional Snacks	Beverages, e.g., Tea, Coffee, Alcohol
Monday				
Tuesday				

Brian Halvorsen, BDS, LDS RCS

Wednesday				
Thursday				
Friday				
Saturday				
Sunday				

Please enter everything you have eaten. Be completely honest with yourself. Remember that this is to help and advise you to better health. Please enter brand names of foods where applicable.

After analyzing both blood tests and diet sheet results, the nutritional practitioner may want to liaise with the patient's medical practitioner, especially if some of the findings require treatment that the practitioner is not qualified to carry out. If there are no basic medical problems, the nutritionist can make recommendations on any necessary dietary improvements. This will not necessarily just be supplementary vitamins and minerals, but it could relate more to the balance and combination of foods. Many, for instance, eat far too much protein and fat; others could be eating far too much fiber, which is robbing them of essential minerals. From personal experience, the results often surprise me, but this only goes to confirm the vast biochemical individuality of every one of us.

The aim of the counseling will be to modify the patient's dietary habits, not only to make him healthier, but also to suit his lifestyle, social, and economic status, and, of course, his taste. To achieve these aims takes time, and it is wise for the counselor to call the patient back after about six weeks to review progress. Some of the recommended dietary changes may not be suitable, and further modifications may be required.

If the dietary changes have originated from a dental problem, the patient can often see vast improvements in the condition in the mouth within a relatively short period of time, say two to three weeks. The gums may have stopped bleeding, breath may be fresher, and the mouth will generally feel cleaner. In tandem with this will be a newfound vitality, a fresher complexion, healthier hair, and a sense of heightened well-being.

Dietary Guidelines

As with many things in life, one tends to set out with great enthusiasm and good intentions, but reality often intercedes and these resolutions soon weaken. I have listed below a series of simple advice points that I hope will strengthen my patients' resolve and act as a memory jerker. These points also encompass many of the principles that I have been advocating throughout this book:

A Whole Food Diet

The term "whole foods" is very simple; there is nothing cantankerous or off-putting about it. It simply means the following:

- foods that have nothing added or taken away
- foods that are as near to their natural state as possible
- foods that are not processed or refined
- foods that do not contain artificial additives, flavorings,

- colors, or preservatives
- just "whole" foods, as close as possible to how nature intended
- no salt or sugar

Salt

Recent studies show that the daily salt or sodium requirement for a human being is probably no more than two hundred milligrams a day. This small quantity is available naturally in whole foods alone, in vegetables, meats and fish, fruits and grains, and no one should have to add salt to foods. However, the average amount taken in by most individuals is more than twenty-five times that amount. Salt seems to be at the root of hypertension, one of our most common twentieth-century illnesses. It also upsets the body's water balance. Once you start to omit salt from your cooking, you will soon learn to do without it. Use fresh and dried herbs, garlic, and spices for seasoning instead.

Sugar

Refined sugar is a totally unnatural substance that has been stripped of any nutritional value. Sugar in concentrated form creates stressful bio-chemical reactions, for example in the pancreas, where an overproduction of insulin can rapidly lower blood sugar levels and consequently a depletion of your energy levels. If this occurs on a frequent basis over a period of time, this may then result in an artificial imbalance which can, in some cases, trigger the onset of diabetes. In England, during World War II (1939–1945), the incidence of new cases of diabetes fell dramatically. It was no coincidence that there was a great shortage of white sugar and the populace lived on homegrown vegetables. As soon as sugar became freely available again, the incidence of diabetes rose to prewar levels and beyond. Is this a coincidence? I think not. Also think of your teeth! Use small amounts of honey and molasses to sweeten your food.

Fiber

This is an important factor in the diet, but if you eat a good whole food diet, you will be eating enough. Consuming wholemeal bread with plenty of salads and vegetables is the correct way of providing nature's own filler.

Additives

Try to avoid whenever possible. These include colorings, preservatives, and flavorings.[114] Preservatives keep normally perishable food fresh long after it should have gone stale, a convenience for manufacturers. Colorings and flavorings are only needed because many people have come to expect them. If food needs disguising to make it taste good, wouldn't you do better without it?

Vitamins and Minerals

Plenty of vitamins and minerals are present in foods like wholemeal bread and pasta, brown rice, and other whole grains, as well as beans, pulses, nuts, and fresh fruits and vegetables. As much as possible, you should try to eat your food either raw or lightly cooked. Processing and overcooking destroys valuable vitamins and minerals needed to keep your body healthy.

Meat and Dairy

You don't need to cut meat from your diet unless you want to! But it is wise to limit your intake of red meat to one or two meals a week. Many people object to the way livestock is reared in modern-

---

114 (a) "Food Additives—What you always wanted to know about food additives but had no one to ask." NAC © 1997–2005. http://www.nac.allergyforum.com/additives/
(b) Hanssen, M. "E for Additives: The Complete E Number Guide." New York: HarperCollins, 1987.

day conditions. One alternative is to choose produce that has been reared in organic and free-range conditions. Always use organic free-range eggs, for example. Milk, cheese, and butter should always be organic, as the fat content will otherwise concentrate pesticide residues, etc.

Organic Food

Good health and good food start in the soil. If soil is deficient, then so is the food grown in it. Deficient crops don't grow properly and are prone to disease and pest attacks. The farming industry's answer is to add pesticides, chemicals, and nitrogenous fertilizers. The result is food full of harmful residue. In addition, foods are sprayed with chemicals so that they stay fresh longer in shops and supermarkets. Some of the vegetables we buy have been sprayed up to forty-seven times! Always wash any vegetables well and try to grow your own or buy organically grown produce when possible. Remember, imported organic food may well be healthier, but it is also likely to be sprayed with preservatives and antifungals, etc., so wash thoroughly before eating. If organic produce is difficult to obtain, locally grown produce such as obtained at farmers' markets makes a good alternative.

Food Wrapping

Any food that is wrapped in plastic is likely to be contaminated with toxic chemicals such as dioxin and DEHA (diethylhexyl). When plastic dissolves, it gives off estrogenic esters. These compounds have been linked to hormone imbalances in humans.[115]

---

115 (a) Plastic Wrap 101. October 4, 2007. http://mindfulmomma.typepad.com/mindful_momma/2007/10/plastic-wrap-10.html
(b) Hahn, J. "A Bad Wrap for Microwaving Food." http://www.seattlepi.com/hahn/53594_hahn08.shtml
(c) "Irish Pigs were fed bread still in plastic bags." *Times Online*, December 7, 2008. http://www.timesonline.co.uk/tol/news/world/europe/article5303184.ece

Planning Your Healthy Diet

Breakfast

People often say they can't face breakfast, but you should try. A good breakfast gives a good start to the day and avoids the eleven o'clock slump that has you reaching for the dreaded doughnut. Muesli is probably the most valuable breakfast food, but others are fresh fruit, oatmeal (use skim milk to keep fat intake down), natural yogurt, wholemeal toast with honey or jam (made with no added sugars or artificial sweeteners), poached or boiled free-range eggs, or compote of dried fruit.

Drink fresh orange juice, herbal or green tea (there are many so experiment until you find one you like), decaffeinated coffee, or mineral water.

Lunch

Our favorite lunch is homemade soup with wholemeal bread. Purée lightly cooked vegetables with stock—nothing could be simpler—or use pulses, like lentils or split peas. Try to have a good helping of salad as well (or have it on its own). Make sure it contains a wide selection of leaf and root vegetables, sprouted seeds, and/or fruit.

Evening Meal

Make your main meal a protein one. Choose from lean meat, fish, poultry, free-range eggs, cheese, or a combination of plant foods, nuts, grains, or pulses. Serve your meal with a raw vegetable salad or lightly steamed vegetables. Include leafy green vegetables. Finish with fresh fruit, yogurt, or a small amount of low-fat cheese.

Drinks for Lunch and Dinner

Try mineral water (check the salt content), a coffee substitute, fresh fruit, or vegetable juices (try making your own; it's worth investing in a juicer). If drinking alcohol, restrict yourself to two glasses of red wine daily and avoid spirits, or have the equivalent in real ale or dry cider. Again, any drinks that are organically produced will be healthier.

Steps toward Healthier Eating

Two nutritional gurus who have been a huge influence on my healthy eating philosophy since the early 1970s are Elizabeth and Curtis Shears. Their dietary principles remain unchallenged for over thirty-five years, and I have outlined some of them below.

The following may seem like a radical regime, but the health benefits will reward your efforts. Empty your larder of all packets and cans of processed and additive-laden foods to avoid temptation. Don't give them to your friends; rubbish belongs in one place only.[116]

Never put off until tomorrow what you can do today. It's not too late to make a start, especially where your health is concerned. The principles below may appear somewhat strict, but by using even some of these nutritional suggestions, the improvement in your physical and mental well-being will spur you on to a greater commitment to healthy eating.

Store Cupboard or Larder Ingredients:

- Where possible, replace all refined and processed foods by 100 percent live whole foods. Especially avoid white flour products.

- Replace all white sugar with molasses and molasses sugar when cooking, and with organic unheated honey when not cooking. All sugars should be used infrequently and in small amounts.

- Replace table, cooking, and sea salt with kelp and occasionally Biosalt (biochemically balanced mineral salt compound).

---

[116] (a) Shears, C. *Nutrition Science and Health Education*. Marlboro: Nutritional Sci. Research Inst of England, 1978.
(b) Shears, E. *Why Do We Eat?* Marlboro: Nutritional Sci. Research Inst of England, 1976

- Replace butter and saturated heated fats and margarines with unheated polyunsaturated margarines and cold pressed vegetable oils such as sunflower, safflower, and olive.

- Replace chocolate with carob or cocoa powder.

- Replace baking soda/baking powder, cream of tartar, and sodium bicarbonate (bicarbonate of soda) with free-range eggs, fresh lemon juice, and plenty of fresh air obtained by sufficient beating or whisking.

- Remove the pepper and salt cruet and replace with three saltshakers, one filled with paprika, one with kelp powder, and the other with brewer's yeast.

- Have available seeds, nuts, and dried fruits if a meal has been missed or for the children when they come home from school. Sunflower seeds are tasty and nutritious.

Produce:

- When cooking vegetables, remember the following principles: eat the flowers, broccoli, cauliflower, purple sprouting broccoli, etc., raw whenever possible; eat the stems and leaves very lightly cooked; and eat the roots cooked a little more (except carrots, which should always be eaten raw). Cook potatoes in their skins.

- Eat the leaves of root vegetables, e.g., beetroot, turnips, and carrot, etc., in a salad or lightly cooked. Eat the outer green leaves of vegetables.

- Eat fruits and vegetables as fresh as possible to obtain the maximum nutritional value. If stored, keep in a cool, dark place, and leave the roots on lettuces, cabbages, etc.

- Replace food grown by artificial fertilizers by food grown organically or biodynamically.

- Wash all fresh fruit and vegetables if you are doubtful of their origin to remove any possible chemical sprays. Wash all dried fruit to remove possible sulphur dioxide, mineral oils, and grit.

- Avoid soaking fresh fruit and vegetables in water; soluble vitamins will suffer. Avoid cooking wherever possible, as this will reduce the vitamin, mineral, and enzyme content of the food. Cook vegetables in the smallest amount of water or in no water at all. Try steaming them. Err on the undercooked rather than the overcooked side.

- Use oil and lemon juice to prevent oxidation of shredded or diced raw vegetables and green salad. Use lemon or orange juice for freshly cut fruit. Have fresh fruit and a fresh green salad daily.

- Grow sprouts from seeds, grains, and legumes year-round; this does not require a garden. Grow as much food as you can following organic principles.

Meat:

- If you eat meat, buy naturally reared animals. If in doubt, buy fish, game, and free-range poultry. Vitamin K is destroyed by freezing so buy liver fresh, not frozen.

- Do not overcook meat. Overcooked or burnt meat can produce carcinogenic compounds such as polycyclic aromatic hydrocarbons (PAHs) and heterocyclic amines (HAs).

Drinks:

- Replace tea, coffee, and cocoa with nutritious cereal drinks, unsweetened fruit juices, unsalted vegetable juices, and herbal teas.

- Avoid drinking with meals that are based on sound nutrition. Drink an hour before a meal or two hours afterwards to avoid diluting the digestive juices. The one exception to the rule is if you ever have the misfortune to have an oversalted or overly sugared meal. Because this could affect your kidneys, drink with the meal as your only salvation, as this helps flush the kidneys.

- Only drink when you are thirsty. On a diet based on sound nutrition, you will find that very little drinking will be necessary. Most of the food you will be eating will contain a large percentage of water.

Cooking Tips:

- Avoid cooking at temperatures above 100°C (212°F), i.e., the temperature used in a pressure cooker. Magnesium, vitamins C and E, and some other vitamins and minerals, as well as all enzymes, can be destroyed nutritionally by heat. Enzymes begin to be destroyed at temperatures as low as 40°C (104°F). To offset these deficiencies in our cooked food, we must obtain them from raw food.

- Ideally, have two-thirds raw food to one-third cooked food. Consume some raw food at every cooked meal.

- Eat all herbs raw for the full mineral and vitamin content. When adding them to hot food, add them at the end of the cooking.

- Never cook with aluminum pans. Use stainless steel or iron utensils.

Vegetarian:

- If vegetarian, then obtain protein from sprouted seeds, grains and legumes, avocado pears, nuts, free-range eggs, brewer's yeast, soya products, yoghurt and green vegetables.

General:

- Avoid cigarettes, spirits, and drugs.

- Avoid rich and concentrated desserts and cakes, even when made of nutritious ingredients.

- Avoid snacks between meals. This indicates that the quality of main meals is not nutritionally adequate. Sugar-containing snacks are likely to increase the risk of tooth decay and diabetes greatly.

- Avoid eating when tired, emotionally upset, or when in a hurry. The digestive processes will be impaired.

- Do not eat too late in the evening. One should breakfast like a king, lunch like a prince, and sup like a pauper, and the latter should be as early as possible to allow digestion to take place before sleep.

- When feeling unwell, cold, or shivery, or when suffering from a sore throat, avoid eating all foods except fresh fruits and vegetables containing an abundance of vitamin C.

- Thoroughly chew your food so that it is a tasteless pulp that can melt away and does not have to be consciously swallowed. This carries out the first stage of digestion in the mouth, and it prepares the rest of the digestive system and body to absorb the nutrients more efficiently.

- Remember that it is not the amount that we eat, but the amount that we assimilate that nourishes.

CHAPTER TWELVE

Nutrition and Ageing: Detox Your Teeth and Your Body

The Bad News

A hundred years ago, the elderly were revered for their accumulated wisdom, especially in a community or tribal environment. Not so today, for the older we get, the greater the body burden (of toxins) becomes. This, combined with an ageing immune system, means that we are less able to cope with maintaining physical and mental health.

I sincerely believe that a major causative factor in this age degeneration process is the accumulation of toxic metals in our bodies, particularly mercury and lead, both powerful neurotoxins. One of the most commonly increasing age-related diseases is Alzheimer's. Professor Boyd-Haley has shown a link between mercury buildup in the brain and people who have died from Alzheimer's. Dr. Gary Gordon has spent many years of his career investigating the link between toxic metals and disease.[117]

Modern man has been exposed to these toxic elements for many years. Current evidence shows[118] that we have one thousand times the lead levels in our bones than our preindustrialized ancestors.

A significant number of studies, both past and present, illustrate the degree to which our environment is polluted by all kinds of toxic chemicals. Through industrialization, intensive agriculture, the

---

117 (a) Alzheimer's—The Diseases http://www.whale.to/d/alzheimers.html
(b) Dr. Garry Gordon, World Leader in Oral Chelation Therapy: http://www.gordonresearch.com/

118 (a) McNamara, L. "Lead In Our Food?" http://ezinearticles.com/?Lead-in-Our-Food?--Now,-THAT-is-a-Heavy-Meal!&id=1273476
(b) Homeopathy Medicine: Detox Programs http://www.yourhealthis.com/homeopathy/index.html

burning of fossil fuels, and other modern life processes, our land, air, and water have all been contaminated to some extent.

The everyday functions of breathing, eating, drinking, and bathing are sufficient to accumulate toxins. Besides lead and mercury, cadmium, aluminium, and arsenic tend to build up in the body rather than be excreted; that is, the older we are, the more we accumulate toxic heavy metals. If you have any doubts about the toxic effects that dental amalgam (50 percent mercury) has on the environment and personal health, use the Internet and search "dental amalgam" and/or "mercury." Look for comments from the World Health Organization (WHO) and Professor Boyd-Haley, to name just two.

It is difficult to distinguish science from nonscience, especially on the Internet. My advice is to take a common sense view of all the information, and where comments such as "scientists have shown" occur, find out whom they are; their motivation; and who is paying for the research.

In January 2008, Norway banned the use of amalgam (mercury) for dental fillings, not just on environmental grounds but also because of their toxic effects on our bodies.[119]

Mercury [Hg] can be found in numerous everyday sources; it is not limited to dental amalgams.

    Sources of mercury:[120]

    Adhesives[121]
    Air conditioner filters
    All fish (in particular, salmon and tuna)

---

119 (a) Miller, A. "Norway Becomes First Country to Ban Amalgam Filling," April 4 2008. http://www.naturalnews.com/022943.html
(b) "Norway, Sweden and Denmark Ban Mercury Amalgams For Environmental and Health Reasons," November 5, 2008. http://www.healthymuslim.com/articles/pvbwj-norway-sweden-anddenmark-ban-mercury-amalgams-for-environmental-and-health-reasons.cfm
120 Source: Gordon Research Institute, Phoenix, Arizona, USA.
121 "Less Toxic Home Repair and Construction Materials." http://www.pollutioninpeople.org/safer/products/buildingmaterials

Animal and industrial waste
Automobile exhausts
Batteries
Body powders (calomel)
Cinnabar (used in jewellery)
Cosmetics
Dental amalgams
Drinking and well water
Fabric softeners
Fertilizers
Floor wax
Hemorrhoid supplements
Laxatives
Paints and pigments
Pesticides
Processed foods
Seafood, seawater
Skin lightening creams
Thimerosal (preservative in medical injections)
Vaccines (as above—many believe the mercury in the MMR vaccine may be linked to autism)
Wood preservatives

It is important to know that even under "normal" environmental and dietary conditions, there is a considerable risk of mercury contamination.

The U.S. Environmental Protection Agency states that the safe limits for mercury vapor exposure are ten micrograms per day. Numerous studies have shown that mercury amalgam fillings release anywhere from one to twenty-nine micrograms per day—up to three times the limit—just for one amalgam!

Average human daily doses of mercury from various sources:*

Mercury Source	Daily Exposure	Form
Dental amalgam	3.0–17.0 micrograms/day	Mercury vapor
Fish/seafood	2.3 micrograms/day	Methyl Mercury
Other food	0.3 micrograms/day	Inorganic Mercury

* These amounts would be increased for persons working with mercury, such as dentists, those who have more than one tooth amalgam, or persons particularly fond of eating fish.

The rate of mercury release from amalgams is dependent upon several factors, including the number of amalgam restorations, the composition of the amalgam (high versus low copper amalgam), the location factors (occusal versus nonocclusal), and the amalgam surface area.[122]

When mercury has "contaminated" tissues such as our brain or bones, it has a minimum half-life of at least fifteen years (this is if no more is added!). This means that its toxic effects can extend for a long time. In dentistry, there is a continual debate about what the safe levels are. The WHO has stated that there is no safe low level of mercury.

Within the dental profession, the amalgam debate has raged for more than 150 years. There can be no argument that in an increasingly toxic environment, any increase of mercury from amalgam fillings will add to the "body burden." The body burden can be defined as how hard the immune system has to work to maintain health at a cellular level (homeostasis).

Mercury and lead are extremely toxic to nerve tissues, and biologically it seems unfair that a poison like mercury can be easily absorbed and assimilated into our bodies but difficult to eliminate. My analogy is that it's like having your best white suit splashed with dirty grease—easy to do, but very difficult to clean.

I believe the toxicity of mercury and lead makes heavy metals the body's number one enemy. When combined, lead makes mercury

---

[122] World Health Organization, Environmental Health Criteria 118, Inorganic Mercury Sources, Geneva 1991.

one hundred times more toxic.[123] Remember, toxicity can be defined as the amount of a substance required to create cellular change. On this planet, only uranium and plutonium are more toxic than mercury!

At the start of this book, Dr. Price's research was chronologically the last time this planet contained some areas that were unpolluted. Now we live on a toxic planet, e.g., mercury from China's coal-burning power stations has been found in large concentrations in the high Rocky Mountains of the United States!

Many holistic practitioners agree that if a person is over forty years old, exposure to leaded gasoline, mercury, and cadmium (smoking and/or passive smoking) means that there is a high probability of a highly toxic body load.

The Good News

There are many nutritional regimes designed to reduce heavy metal buildup in the body. Prevention is better than cure, so following a safe, well-balanced diet will reduce the likelihood of age-related disease.

Dr. Brian's Diet to Reduce Your Intake of Toxins/Heavy Metals:

1. Eat organically grown produce whenever possible in order to avoid consuming mercury from fungicides and pesticides.

2. Avoid eating large amounts of tuna and swordfish, which may contain unacceptable levels of mercury. Instead, stick mainly to deepwater fish such as cod, haddock, and sole. For omega-3 fatty acids, consume smaller oily fish such as sardines and mackerel.

---

123 Synergistic Toxicity. http://www.whale.to/vaccine/synergistic_toxicity_q.html

3. Eat at least five portions of organic fresh fruits and vegetables each day.

4. Choose a variety of colors for their antioxidant pigment and carotenoids, a class of natural fat-soluble pigments responsible for many of the red, orange, and yellow colors found in plants.[124]

5. Consume plenty of vegetables from the *Brassica* family, e.g., brussels sprouts, broccoli, cauliflower, cabbages, etc. These foods increase the activity of the phase II glutathione S-transferase system, which helps detoxify heavy metals. Sulphur contained in these vegetables chelates heavy metals.[125]

6. Eat plenty of foods containing soluble fiber, particularly pectin, which binds to toxins and draws them from the body. Good fiber foods include natural grains, brown rice, oatmeal, millet, corn, and flaxseed; note that these also contain good levels of B vitamins, which act as cofactors for liver enzyme systems.

7. Do not consume refined sugars, as they drive mercury into the cell rather than allowing it to exit the body through its natural route—the bowel. Eat fresh fruit instead.

8. Drink less beer, spirits, and white wine. Red wines contain potent antioxidants, so the occasional glass is acceptable, but remember that alcohol inhibits the natural detoxification pathways in the body.

9. Consume members of the onion family regularly. These vegetables are rich in sulphur compounds to increase liver

---

[124] Carotenoids http://www.astaxanthin.org/carotenoids.htm
[125] Graham King, Guy Barker: "Health, Medical, and Clinical benefits of Brassica consumption," HRI-Wellesbourne. November 2003. http://www.brassica.info/info/crop-enduses/nutritional-benefits.php

sulphation, which is used to back up the glutathione detox system.

10. Eat many selenium-rich foods—seeds and nuts, particularly walnuts—because selenium is required to bind mercury and inactivate it.

11. Reduce the intake of hydrogenated fats that are often found in margarine, cookies, and sweet snacks. Instead, eat plenty of polyunsaturated fats found in borage seeds, olive oil, hemp seeds, sunflower seeds, grape seeds, sesame seeds, and avocados. Also cut down the consumption of saturated fats, e.g., those found in sausages, burgers, and canned meat. Plus, avoid trans fats—those found in crisps, chips, and food fried in polysaturated fats.

12. Avoid artificial flavors, colors, and preservatives. Many will add to your "toxic burden," so your body will work harder to detox heavy metals, etc.

13. Avoid caffeine—it's a potent diuretic (including decaffeinated coffee!), increases toxin accumulation, and is a potent toxin (caffeine hydrochloride).[126]

14. Stop smoking and avoid smoky atmospheres (cadmium exposure).

15. Avoid polluted regions.

16. Drink plenty of hydrating fluids, e.g., spring, mineral, or filtered water, as opposed to diuretic drinks such as coffee, tea, and colas.

---

126 (a) "E Numbers, Food Additives, Preservatives, Toxins, Colors, Health." http://curezone.com/foods/enumbers.asp
(b) Whalen, R. "Dangers of Caffeine, with References." http://www.doctoryourself.com/caffeine2.html

NB: The last six tips will reduce the total load on the liver, paramount to allowing maximum detoxification of mercury, lead, and cadmium to take place.

Modifications can be made to this program to suit the individual.

To achieve maximum benefit from a chelating/detox diet, consult a well-trained nutritionist. Look for nutritional therapists who have trained in whole food nutrition and who follow a holistic approach with their clients.

Supplements—a Twenty-First-Century Way to Avoid the Diseases of Ageing?

How many times has it been stated that if you eat a well-balanced diet, you shouldn't need supplements? My question is: "If we are having this 'well-balanced diet,' why are so many people suffering and dying from nutritionally linked diseases?"

In my area of special interest, i.e., dental health, there is a graphic example of poor diet being directly linked to the most common diseases in the world—tooth decay and gum disease!

As I have indicated, the mouth can be seen as a barometer of health for the whole body, so it follows that nutrition that benefits the body will also benefit the teeth and gums and vice versa.

Let's be real. We cannot return to the pre–Weston Price era and live the lifestyle of the isolated primitives existing on nourishing diets. Although we can try not to, most of us will include in our diets, to a lesser or greater extent, processed convenience foods. The reasons are numerous, including the expense and availability of organic or locally grown produce. Also, it is often difficult to obtain healthy food when eating out or travelling.

For these and many other reasons, including combating pollution, taking the correct supplements can provide us all with some "health insurance." Just as specific nutrients can prevent a particular disease process, there are minerals, vitamins, enzymes, coenzymes, fatty acids, trace elements, etc., that nutritional science has shown, if taken in the correct quantity, combination, and balance, will improve our health and well-being.

Because we are all biochemically unique, our supplement regime will also differ. Your requirements will also be different if you are a growing child, or during menopause or puberty, and even whether you are a man or a woman!

Supplements and Gum Disease

Over the last thirty years, I have often noticed that despite good dental hygiene and regular visits to the hygienist, some of my patients suffer a decline in their gum health. On questioning, most will admit to "stress overload"; this is not age related but an accumulation of life stresses (see the Four Stresses on page 172). In these circumstances, I will often recommend large doses of vitamin C.

My patients with gum problems will often say, "But I eat plenty of fruit and vegetables, so why do I need more vitamin C?" Note that the minimal dose of one thousand milligrams is equivalent to forty fresh oranges! At this dosage, there is little risk of overdosage, as any excess just passes through the body. However, at this dosage and above, vitamin C is proactively helping the body fight gum disease.

It is important that a practitioner knows the patient's medical history and only prescribes supplements that are safe, or consults with the patient's doctor if there is any possibility of adverse reactions.

Have a look at Dr. Linus Pauling's book *Vitamin C and the Common Cold*, in which this chemist—twice Nobel Prize winner—advocates taking large doses of vitamin C daily to protect against colds and improve general health by building body resistance and thus reducing susceptibility to infections. What is good for the body is good for the gums and vice versa.

Over the years, many hundreds of my patients have benefited from taking regular large doses of vitamin C.

Many clinical trials have shown the effectiveness of Coenzyme Co Q10 in reducing gum disease.[127] Again, the mode of action of Q10 is by boosting the immune system. Q10 is manufactured naturally in the liver but declines with age. Effective dosage tends to be in the region of 100mg per day. Q10 appears to be extremely safe with little if any side effects.

I have found that vitamin C and Q10 work well together to improve gum health; however, many patients report other improvements in their general health.

Another common condition, recurrent mouth ulcers, also responds well to large doses of vitamin C (at least one thousand milligrams per day). If vitamin C is not completely effective, then daily amounts of zinc (thirty to fifty milligrams) usually do the trick.

The above are specific to holistic dental practice and can be administered safely.

Chelation

When we enter the specific area of using supplements for detoxing/chelation,[128] my strong recommendation to my patients is that they be under the care of an experienced nutrition practitioner, preferably with a medical background. Although there are many well-formulated supplements, we are all individuals, so great care is required when considering a chelation program. Remember, "One man's meat is another man's poison" says it all.

---

127 (a) Co-Enzyme Q10. http://www.vitaminsuk.com/index.php?main_page=articles&topic=coenzymeq10
(b) Co-Enzyme Q10. http://www.healthandgoodness.com/acatalog/Coenzyme_Q10.html
128 Detoxification Explained. http://prohealtharticle.com/2009/01/17/detoxification-explainedways-to-detox-your-body-during-a-weight-loss-program/

Conclusion

Where Do I See the Future of Holistic Dentistry/Medicine?

By combining the accumulation of medical wisdom with biophysical/energetic medicine, holistic practitioners of all specialties can work together for the benefits of their patients.

As human beings, we are slowly realizing that our thoughts have the ability to achieve anything from healing to creating miracles. Over my years as a practitioner, I have witnessed many of my patients recovering from terminal illness and devastating tragedies through a combination of willpower and lifestyle changes.

Quantum physics can now give scientific "meat" to therapies such as applied kinesiology, homeopathy, and various forms of healing and acupuncture. (See *It's the Thought That Counts* by David R. Hamilton.)

My passion is to improve the quality of people's lives. Correct nutrition from before birth to old age gives us all the best potential to achieve this.

Having a polluted brain and body reduces our chances of achieving a quality old age. I believe we have a duty to ourselves to maintain optimum health. Consider taking the correct supplements, reading self-improvement books, and trying meditation and soul-body-mind exercises such as yoga. These all provide "health insurance" for us all.

Abundance, health, and happiness,
Brian Halvorsen

FURTHER READING

Advice to the Reader

I strongly suggest that you do not accept everything I have written! Instead, check out any areas of the contents that you might find difficult to believe or simply want to know more about. We are entering the Age of Aquarius, where more and more of us want the truth about what we are told. On the Web, most controversial subjects will have plants, i.e., Web sites deliberately designed to mislead. An example is "'Too Much Vitamin C is Harmful." When you visit such sites, consider the following:

- Does it make sense from your own experience?
- Who are the so-called "scientists" who are making these claims? Have they spent their whole careers on that subject? Who funded the project?
- "Show me the science" (motto of the IAOMT)
- Read *Power Vs. Force* by David Hawkins. You will then be able to distinguish between truth and falsehood.

The Internet is a fantastic way of linking us all, and if used with the right intentions, it will benefit mankind. *Beware of the pollution.*

Brian Halvorsen

Selected Bibliography from the 1986 Book *The Natural Dentist*

[Please note that this list was part of the original 1986 book, edited by Gale Reebok, now CEO and Chairman of Random House Group, and that many of these books are now out of print or relatively unavailable.]

- John Besford. *Good Mouthkeeping*. Debeli Press, 1980.

- Geoffrey Cannon and Caroline Walker. *The Food Scandal.* Century, 1985.
- R. A. Cawson. *Essentials of Dental Surgery and Pathology.* Churchill Livingstone, 1978.
- Cooper Products. Current Aspects of Dental Health. 1983.
- Cowell and Sheihan. *Promoting Dental Health.* King Edwards Hospital Fund, Pitman Books, 1981.
- Dr. C. Curtis Shears. *Nutritional Science and Health Education.* Castle Press, 1974.
- John Forrest. *The Good Teeth Guide.* Granada, 1981.
- Doris Grant. *Fluoridation and the Forgotten Issue.* National Anti-Fluoridation Campaign.
- Harold Gelb and Paula M. Siegel. *Killing Pain Without Prescription.* Thorsons, 1983.
- Miranda Hall. *Feeding Your Children.* Piatkus Books, 1984.
- Maurice Hansson. *E for Additives.* Thorsons, 1985.
- Walter Hoffman-Anthelm. *History of Dentistry.* Quintessence Publishing Co., 1981
- G. Neil Jenkins. *The Physiology and Biochemistry of the Mouth.* Blackwell Scientific Publications, 1978.
- Dr. Hugh Jolly. *The Book of Child Care.* Sphere, 1981.
- Leslie and Susannah Kenton. *Raw Energy.* Century, 1984.
- Penelope Leach. *Baby and Child.* Penguin, 1982.
- Lilian Lindsay. *A Short History of Dentistry.* John Bale, Sons, and Danielsson Ltd, 1933.
- Shklar McCarthy. *The Oral Manifestations of Systemic Disease.* Butterworths, 1976.
- J D. Manson. *Periodontics.* Henry Kimpton, 1966.
- Dr. Weston Price. *Nutrition and Physical Degeneration.* Price-Pottenger Foundation, 1970.
- Herman Prinz. *Dental Chronology.* Henry Kimpton, 1945.
- Patricia M. Randolph and Carol I. *Dennison, Diet, Nutrition and Dentistry.* The C. V. Mosby Company, 1981.
- Elizabeth Shears. *Why Do We Eat?* Mulberry Press, 1976.
- Dr. Sheldon B Sidney. *Ignore Your Teeth and They'll Go Away.* Devida Publications, 1982.
- Drs. Penny and Andrew Stanway. *Breast Is Best.* Pan, 1978.

- G. C. Van Beek. *Dental Morphology.* Wright Publishing Co., 1983.
- John Woodforde. *The Strange Story of False Teeth.* Tandem, 1968.
- Professor John Yudkin. *Pure, White and Deadly.* Davis-Poynter Ltd, 1972.
- Sam Ziff. *The Toxic Time Bomb.* Aurora Press, 1984.

Additional References for *Great Teeth for Life*

Association for the Promotion of Preconceptual Care. Web site: www.foresight-preconception.org.uk
British Dental Health Foundation (BDHF). Web site: www.dentalhealth.org.uk
USA Dental Health Foundation. Web site: www.dentalhealthfoundation.org
The American Academy of Periodontology. Web site: www.perio.org
Acidogenicity of Common Snack Foods, W. M. Edgar and reproduced from Diet, *Nutrition & Dentistry* by Randolph and Dennison (The Mosby Company 1981)
Brian Halvorsen. Email: brian@greatteethforlife.com
Brian Halvorsen. Web site: www.greatteethforlife.com
Amalgam Information. Web site: www.amalgam.org
Antiaging Magazine. Web site: www.antiaging-magazine.com
British Dental Association (BDA). Web site: www.bda.org.uk
Cosmetic Results. Web site: www.dental-picture-show.com/cosmetic_dentistry/a1_smile_makeovers.html
Cosmetic Techniques. Information: http://en.wikipedia.org/wiki/Cosmetic_dentistry
HealOzone. Web site: www.dentalzone.co.uk
Healthy Nutrition. Web site: www.price-pottenger.org
International Academy of Oral Medicine & Toxicology, IAOMT. Web site: www.iaomt.org
"It's the Thought that Counts" by David R. Hamilton PhD. Hay House.
Mercury and Autism. Web site: www.thelastoutpost.com
Mercury and CFS/ME. Web site: www.beatcfsandfms.org
Mercury and MS. Web site: www.msrc.co.uk
Mercury Exposure. Web site: www.mercuryexposure.org
Metal Allergy Blood Tests. Web site: www.melisa.org
Zoom Whitening. Web site: www.zoomnow.com

Beyond Diet and Lifestyle

Why Supplements Are an Essential Part of the Detoxification Process

By Phil Micans, MS, PharmB

I first came across Dr. Brian Halvorsen about ten years ago, when I sought him out to remove my own dental amalgams, which had been deposited there by the school-visiting dentists, people who had been encouraged to do something to everyone they saw, since they only got paid by drilling, filling, and billing.

But with Dr. Halvorsen, I soon discovered that he was one of the few dental practitioners in the United Kingdom who was not only interested in removing my amalgams, but also someone who understood the need to do so, and what additional requirements were necessary to continue to reduce and remove the toxins from my mouth and body.

In other words, Dr. Halvorsen was aware of the issues and wanted to do something about them. As my background is biochemistry and pharmacy, and with my knowledge of what was available on the global market (in terms of effective products and some of my connections to experts in the field such as Garry Gordon, MD), this soon meant that we struck up both a professional relationship as well as a friendship.

Dentistry

Indeed, Dr. Halvorsen and I have worked together to help improve the condition and the environment for dentists and their assistants. The fact that so many people want their amalgams removed, to be replaced with more aesthetically pleasing white types (that don't use mercury and silver) means that dentists and their staff are exposing themselves to massive amounts of mercury vapor.

You may remember the old saying "mad as a hatter" (which was a theme in the famous book *Alice in Wonderland*). It came about because hatters of old used mercury in the steam to shape the hats. As a consequence of breathing it in themselves, they became senile early. Of course, those practices were halted many years ago, but take a guess at which profession is at the highest risk of Alzheimer's disease today? Who could be regularly breathing in mercury vapors? That's right—dentists.

There have already been lawsuits in America, where dental assistants (who often don't even wear masks) have sued their employers as a result of their own problems, or the problems of their newborn children, relating them to the toxic environment of the dental office.

This issue is going to have a major impact on dental practices in many countries over the coming years. Currently, the vast majority of practices offer no advice, little protection against contamination, and certainly no methods to chelate mercury for their employees.

Micro-mercurialism

Of course, a dementia is a very serious consequence of mercury contamination, but there are many other symptoms related to smaller levels of accumulation. Note I did not use the word toxicity, as that implies a higher level of accumulation, but depending upon the amount, the individual's hypersensitivity to it, and the positioning of the mercury molecules—in particular membranes—the outcome can be different for each individual.

According to Dr. Dietrich Klinghardt of the University of Geneva in Switzerland, all of the symptoms listed in the following table are associated with micro-mercurialism.

Allergies	Alzheimer's	Anger
Anxiety	Appetite loss	Autism
Autoimmune diseases	Bleeding gums	Cardiac irregularity
Constipation	Depression	Excessive sweating
Facial pain	Fatigue	Gait problems
GI complaints	Hair loss	Hallucinations

Headaches	Hearing disorders	High emotions
Hormone imbalances	Indigestion	Insomnia
Irritability	Joint pain and inflammation	Kidney function impairment
Libido reduction	Loss of confidence	Lupus
Memory problems	Migraines	Multiple Sclerosis
Muscle pain and weakness	Nervousness	Numb lips and feet
Periodontal disease	Poor dusk vision	Seizures
Skin inflammation	Speech disorders	Subclinical hypothyroidism
Stomatitis	Stool problems	Tinnitus
Tremors	Twitching	Urinary problems
Vertigo	Weight gain	Yeast injections

People need to be aware of these facts. That is why I am delighted that Dr. Halvorsen has written *Great Teeth For Life*, as it is a much-needed appraisal of the potential health issues associated with dentistry and our contaminated world at large.

I am sure that we all agree that avoidance and prevention is the key, but it is extremely difficult to be 100 percent "clean" in our modern world; in fact, I would say it is impossible.

As such, Dr. Halvorsen has asked me to add a little something to the book, giving some information about which supplements can help, and I am delighted to be able to do so.

Practicality

I lost my front teeth in a rugby accident, and since my mid-twenties, I have been stuck with two metal posts in my gums. I'm aware of the heavy metal issue of these posts, but as I don't want to seem like an inane idiot every time I smile, I have to accept the reality and be aware of the problem. In order to be practical, I chelate and detox myself regularly; this can be a lot easier than it sounds once one has gotten into a routine.

Food and lifestyle are obviously a great place to start, and they should form the basis of everyone's basic foundation of health. I think it is a great benefit for all to understand more about how food can detox us; clearly this goes beyond the taste and nutrition factors of food, details of which bombard us from our television sets. Therefore, it's a credit that Dr. Halvorsen's book has details about the chelation properties of different foodstuffs, which we can all use every day.

We are challenged by the continuous absorption of toxins, whether through dental procedures or industrial contaminants in the food chain and air, and the fact that organic food today is considerably depleted in terms of its nutritional qualities compared to that of fifty years ago. Without even mentioning the many nutritionally poor processed foods we consume, we can realize that there is an argument to go beyond diet and lifestyle.

Why Bother?

The evidence being amassed about the dangers of heavy metal toxicity is overwhelming. When you understand the pressures behind the scenes, you understand why the authorities are so slow to respond to things; in my opinion, it's a case of hearing it from them last.

It's akin to the reasoning behind why a "safe" cigarette was never introduced, when it could have been. If such an action was to occur, then it becomes an admission that the previous ones were dangerous and ergo opens the door to a slew of lawsuits.

The positioning behind metals in dentistry being safe, particularly mercury, is becoming more difficult to maintain, and especially since countries like Norway are banning it on health grounds, the landslide of the change of the "official position" has begun.

You can see from the Dr. Klinghardt's list that mercury has been linked with many nasty problems, and the combination of other heavy metals, particularly lead, creates negative synergy. In other words, the detrimental effects of these metals on our systems increases when they are found in combination, thus this is not just a simple case of the physical amounts of these metals that can be found in our bodies.

Meanwhile, the population at large is suffering from an explosion of dementias; the older we become, the more likely we are to develop one of the forms of dementia. It could be that over the age of eighty, only one in seven do not have a dementia! With an ever-increasing ageing population, how are we going to overcome, or at least significantly reduce, this problem? Long-term chelation is one possible answer.

At the other end of the age scale, we have some worrying statistics about our children. For example, autism, which has been related to mercury exposure (and this includes that from vaccines) and used to affect 1 in 10,000 children in 1970, rose to 1 in 166 in the late 1990s. In March 2004, the American Academy of Pediatrics issued an "alarm" to pediatricians across America, warning that autism is "prevalent and must be treated early."

In fact, the U.S. Department of Education data suggests that the rates of autism between 1992 and 2002 are up 1000 percent in all states.

The combination of poor nutrition, changes in lifestyle and exercise, loss of family values and supporting social structures, plus the varying issues of toxicity, now account for the belief by some specialists, such as Dr. Garry Gordon, that by the age of six, only one in four children is neurologically well developed! Read that again, just in case you missed it: one in four is brain healthy; three out of four are not ...

It's not a pleasant thought, but the reality is that the body likes to keep itself in equilibrium, so it will dump its toxins into what it perceives as new tissue; a developing baby is new tissue, in the same way as is a cancer growth! One of the reasons that cancer seems to develop and proliferate quickly could well be due to the higher content of toxins and heavy metals passed to the tumor from other parts of the body.

While we are thinking outside the box, how many times have you heard about an elderly person who takes a fall, breaking a major bone (let us say the hip), and is then bedbound in hospital? Then, several weeks later, you hear the news that Aunty May is dead; she died of pneumonia in the hospital, end of story, or so most people accept. I would say that this is a relatively well-known scenario.

Yet Aunty May most probably died of lead poisoning! You see, the bones are a major storage point of heavy metals, particularly lead. Bone cells take many years to turn over (on average, seven years, compared to months for most other cells in the body), thus bone has a problem removing toxins from itself, and the toxins become somewhat "trapped" in them.

So when Aunty May broke her hip, she started releasing massive amounts of those heavy metals straight into her blood—remember that the body likes to keep things in equilibrium. Lead is well known to inhibit the activity of blood cells, so once the balance is tipped, then immunity begins to fail. Accordingly, with a shattered immune system as well as her hip, Aunty May was then predisposed to the first nasty bug that came along (and a hospital is a good place to find them), hence she died of pneumonia, and that was listed on her death certificate—yet lead toxicity triggered the chain of events that led (pun intended) to her demise.

Chelation can also make sense in another unusual way; some consider it the most potent antioxidant ever. Yet most of the supplements used for chelation are poor free radical scavengers in themselves, so how can these two statements be true? The answer is that most free radicals are generated in the presence of heavy metals; for example, iron and lead molecules in the skin react with the UV from sunlight to become vicious free radicals. The typical results of this action lead to sun-damaged skin, wrinkles (so-called photoaging), and cancer. Experiments have shown that reduction of metals in skin content allows individuals to sunbathe for longer without burning and reduces the risk of the appearance of sun spots (hence cancer). Plus, for those with aesthetics on their mind, this also means a significantly reduced risk for the formation of wrinkles.

The bottom line is, the fewer heavy metals there are in your body, the lower the potential incidences of free radical generations become. Beyond this, there is mounting evidence that heavy metals are behind many disease processes, including arteriosclerosis, blood pressure, cardiovascular, renal failure, cataract, and even cancers, and that by lowering the quantity of heavy metals in the body, that in turn this can improve the condition (some examples are given).

One of the prime uses of chelation therapy is to clear out the arteries, particularly with substances such as EDTA (see the A–Z list below), as it helps to remove calcium plaques. This action not only improves vital blood flow capabilities, but it also softens the arterial wall. These actions ultimately improve the heart condition, partly by not having to make it work as hard to pump blood through hard and constricted arteries.

EDTA has been used for decades in literally hundreds of thousands of patients, primarily for the purposes of clearing out arteries and improving the cardiovascular condition. In one study of 24,000 patients, 88 percent of them exhibited clinical improvement with EDTA therapy; another study of 2,870 patients saw excellent improvement to 90 percent of the patients undertaking the EDTA therapy.

Despite the fact that the average doctor has not heard about EDTA, there are literally stacks of published information about it in the medical journals.

There are many good reasons to chelate and detox, and I've only mentioned a few of them.

Chelating Supplements

So, what are these special chelating supplements? Which ones can provide that extra boost—to kick-start a detox program, to focus on a particular need, to cleanse oneself for fertility and pregnancy purposes (and I refer to men as well as women here), or simply make sure that insurance for a long, healthy life is available? I shall list below some of the most prominent natural supplements that can provide that assurance to back up and bolster a good diet and lifestyle.

But in the meantime, let us also remember that just because something may be in a pill or a capsule, that doesn't make it a drug and that we have to be sick to be swallowing it. Super-concentrated extracts of foodstuffs are designer food supplements or, to put it another way, using natural supplements in this way makes one a scientific greengrocer!

A–Z List

Some of the best supplements that have been regularly used to chelate and detox include the following:

Allicin:

Allicin is found in garlic; it is the substance that gives it its distinctive odor. Apart from being a potent natural antibiotic (researchers from the University of East London have successfully treated the so-called "hospital bug," MRSA, with it), allicin is also known to be able to chelate heavy metals, especially lead and mercury.

Studies have shown that the fetal excretions of mercury can increase by as much as 400 percent when allicin is taken regularly.

Di-indolylmethane (DIM):

Di-indolylmethane is the active constituent found inside *Brassica* vegetables such as cabbages, brussels sprouts, cauliflower, and broccoli, etc. DIM helps improve the transferase system within the body to detox heavy metals by helping to get them excreted.

In addition, DIM is also a potent rebalancer and is involved in the excretion of potentially dangerous estrogens, in particular the form known as "estradiol." This is important because pseudo estrogens are leaking into the environment from plastics, pesticides, and other drugs. The WHO recognizes these toxins in the environment and refers to them as "endocrine disruptors"; in other words, changers of hormones.

It has already been noted that many fish and mammalian species have changed sex and had many other problems due to the presence of these estrogen-type substances. In fact, many leading physicians such as Garry Gordon, MD, and Jonathan Wright, MD, are advocating that these estrogens may be responsible for many cancers, in particular cervical, breast, and prostate.

DIM has the potential to both reduce and balance estrogen ratios in the body, and it therefore stands as an important natural substance for supplementation.

DMSA:

DMSA is the abbreviation for dimercaptosuccinic acid. It is also known as succinic acid. It is perhaps the most potent single oral chelator of both mercury and cadmium. In addition, DMSA also shows reasonable affinity for chelating lead and arsenic.

DMSA is often used orally prior to an intravenous chelation therapy, but unless required for acute cases, it is rarely used on a permanent basis. For example, Dr. Gordon himself takes oral DMSA on a one-month-on, one-month-off basis.

EDTA:

EDTA stands for ethylene diamine tetra acetic acid, which is a synthetic amino acid related to vinegar. EDTA is perhaps the most universally used chelator. Once it is inside the body, it binds heavy metals to itself, holding onto them tightly, and then together they are excreted out, most commonly through urine.

EDTA is the chelator most commonly used in the detox clinic, and it is normally administered as an intravenous (IV) drip, which means up to an hour is required for it all to pass into the blood. However,

EDTA can also be used orally (and due to that ease of use, more regularly too). When used orally, EDTA is considered approximately 10 percent as effective as the IV method; nonetheless, EDTA still has a strong action. For example, a report by the Los Alamos Research Laboratory in New Mexico showed that EDTA taken orally excreted five to ten times more lead out of children than placebo alone. This has also been confirmed by the Australian Industrial Hygiene Division. Furthermore, EDTA has also been shown to remove cadmium, aluminium, iron, nickel, and mercury.

As mentioned earlier (under the subtitle "Why Bother?"), one of the principal roles of EDTA has been to remove calcium plagues from arteries, thereby improving blood flow, reducing arterial stiffness, and lessening the "load" on the heart itself.

Note that it is important to only use the calcium version of EDTA (and not the sodium version), and whilst there is some evidence that EDTA does take out some good minerals (zinc, for example), the amounts are small and can easily be compensated by taking a multivitamin/mineral supplement regularly.

Furthermore, EDTA can be used in a number of ways other than IV and orally; for example, it can be chewed in gums to help capture mercury in the mouth, or placed as a powder into bathtubs to help cleanse the skin.

Fiber:

The role of fiber cannot be overlooked in the chelation and detoxification process. This is because whilst other products help to bind and shift toxins from the membranes they are residing in, many find their way to the gut once "released."

In theory, once they have arrived in the gut, some of these toxins may simply accumulate, causing other problems. However, they can be shifted by fiber and passed out of the body; this is a primary action of fiber—to remove toxins from the digestive tract.

Excellent fiber sources include the husks of brown rice and the Jerusalem artichoke. In addition, legumes (beans, peas, and lentils), wheat bran, prunes, acai, raspberries, and blackberries are also good sources of fiber.

L-ascorbic acid:

L-ascorbic acid is the active part of vitamin C. It is important to know if the vitamin C you are taking is listed as L-ascorbic acid because if it is just listed as "ascorbic acid" (or vitamin C), it is likely to contain both the L and D versions, which would mean that the effective dose would be half of what was listed on the label.

L-ascorbic acid has probably had more published studies conducted on it than any other substance. The late Nobel laureate Linus Pauling studied it in depth. He stated that it has the widest range of uses of a vitamin within the body, yet unfortunately it remains the only vitamin that the body cannot store.

Dr. Thomas Levy's book *Vitamin C, Infectious Diseases and Toxins* has numerous studies listed in it that have shown L-ascorbic acid to have chelation abilities in humans. To give you some idea, ascorbic acid has been shown to reduce pesticides, carbon monoxide, arsenic, chromium, cadmium, aluminium, chlorine, and fluoride levels in the body.

Malic acid:

Malic acid is a vital component in the energy-producing Krebs cycle but also has many other important roles in the body, including the maintenance of the acid balance as well as the removal of undesirable metals by chelation; in particular, malic acid is noted for removing lead, aluminium, and strontium.

A good source of malic acid is from apples, which may be one of the reasons why Grandma always said that an apple a day keeps the doctor away!

Selenium:

Selenium is a potent antioxidant found in soil, plants, and fish. The better meats (in terms of selenium quantities) are tuna, cod, beef, and turkey; the better plants are Brazil nuts, oatmeal, and rice (note that whole eggs are also a good source). Selenium assists the body in using vitamin E and has an important role in enzyme and protein synthesis.

This rare trace element binds itself to mercury and essentially deactivates it. This is because once mercury is bound to the selenium it becomes a new molecule that the body cannot absorb. Now, whilst selenium by itself doesn't remove mercury from the body, the fact that it can effectively "silence" its action is an important part of the chelation process.

A good way to think about selenium is to understand that it acts like a mercury magnet. As such, an alternative theory of late is that the mercury seeks out and attaches itself to selenium. In so doing, the mercury prevents the selenium from carrying out in protein and enzyme processes in the body.

This second theory gives an even stronger need to take additional selenium supplements to overcome mercury's actions, particularly since poorer soil conditions for trace elements such as selenium mean that ever-declining intakes are to be obtained from the diet.

Zeolite:

Zeolite is perhaps the "new kid on the block"—that is, if you can call waiting three hundred million years for it to develop *new*! What I mean is that zeolite is a crystal formed from volcanic ash, but in terms of using it for chelation, that purpose is relatively new.

What's interesting about zeolite is that due to its honeycomb shape, it has many "arms" to reach out and grab heavy metals, and what's more, it doesn't appear to grab healthy minerals like zinc, instead passing them by and leaving them in situ.

Zeolite seems to have a fast action too; users often report on the darker color of their urine within an hour or so of ingesting Zeolite, an obvious sign that toxins have been shifted.

Zeolite has been described as being a good chelator for aluminium, arsenic, cadmium, lead, mercury, and tin from the blood and soft tissues, but it may not be as effective for extracting deeper deposited toxins.

The best form of zeolite to use is in a nano-sized sublingual form. A nano molecule is very small indeed, usually expressed in terms of one to one hundred nanometers. A "normal" molecule is expressed in terms of Daltons, and a nano molecule is so much smaller than a Dalton that it has approximately ten times the surface area of a Dalton molecule. Thus, nano molecules are considered more efficient in delivering a more effective dose of a product—in this case, it is particularly true of zeolite.

Synergy, Efficacy, and Quality

I appreciate that the selection above seems like quite a long list, but there are products available today that contain many of these items all in one, thus reducing the inconvenience of having to take dozens of pills regularly.

In the course of my own business, I've been lucky enough not to be stuck with having to sell one particular brand or another. Coming from a research background and having a personal interest in the field (plus wanting the best for my family and myself), I sought out the great researchers and practitioners to see what they were recommending from the scientific and clinical literature. Thus, I have been able to create a unique and diverse selection of supplements—simply put, the best the world has to offer.

I appreciate how difficult it is in the nutritional supplement world to ponder the differences and rationales behind a good product versus an average product, especially since that decision ultimately does take into consideration knowledge of the ingredients, their dosages, their sources, and the integrity of the company itself.

Dr. Gordon's own Beyond range of products is one such example of those from the high-end. Safe in the knowledge that they are designed and formulated by a world expert in chelation, when one also realizes that Dr. Gordon relies upon them for his own health, and when one learns how to read labels, then one realizes they are something special.

A dedication to finding clean, organic sources of materials is the other. I remember Dr. Gordon telling me that he changed his supplier for garlic; the original supplier had been fine, but later testing on batches showed that contaminants were somehow finding their way into the material. A trip to the supplier discovered that a major road had been built alongside the farmland, and naturally the toxic output of the vehicles was finding its way into the plants. Thus, he changed suppliers for a cleaner source.

This type of thing is all part of the battle to live as cleanly as possible on our polluted planet, but hopefully it is a good example of the dedication to the cause to be the best.

At the end of the day, as far as supplements are concerned, it is their synergy, their efficacy, and their quality that separates the best from the rest.

Conclusion

Many supplements are created to fit a budget; only some are designed to meet a standard. Eventually, when you find a quality range of supplements, then you'll understand why you may be paying a bit more for them, but why you will never want to go back to your old "value" brand!

Making your diet and lifestyle changes and incorporating quality, synergistic supplements such as those mentioned above can make significant changes in just weeks to your energy levels, your well-being, and your quality of life.

In the meantime, the gradual release of those heavy metals and toxins from your system will reduce your body's burdens. The net result will be an improved immune system, resulting in dramatically reduced instances of feeling under the weather.

In addition, evidence suggests that there will also be a reduction in the likelihood of the development of numerous so-called age-related diseases and disorders, including reducing the risk of developing a dementia, cardiovascular disease, or cancer.

Chelation and detox is an excellent example of preventative anti-ageing medicine at its best, and one that anyone can introduce to his health program, no matter his current age or condition. Dr. Halvorsen and I know this because we have seen it repeatedly in patients who make such a commitment to a change for the better.

I hope that this book will become your reference guide for a positive change in your and your family's health.

Additional Reading

- *Our Toxic World, A Wake-Up Call* by Doris J. Rapp, MD, published by the Environmental Medical Research Foundation.
- *The Chelation Way* by Dr. Morton Walker, published by Avery.
- *Vitamin C, Infectious Diseases and Toxins* by Thomas E. Levy, MD, published by Xlibris.
- *Toxic Metal Syndromes, How Metal Poisonings Can Affect Your Brain* by Dr. Richard Casdorph, published by Avery.
- *Detox with Oral Chelation, Protecting Yourself From Lead, Mercury, And Other Environmental Toxins* by Garry Gordon, MD, published by Smart Publications.

Index

A
abscesses, 106–107, 132
Abulcasis, 14
acid erosion, 3, 168
acidogenicity of common foods, 101
acid response, 112
acute gum disease, 128–129
acute ulcerative gingivitis (AUG), 23, 128–129
Addis, William, 141
additives, 65, 189
adrenalin, 178
alcohol, 52, 64–65, 70, 170, 192, 202
alfalfa, 77–78
allicin, 220
aluminium, 198, 223
Alzheimer's disease, 173, 175, 197, 214
amalgam fillings, 20, 21, 53, 61–62, 198–200, 213–214
amelogenesis imperfecta, 37
amyloglucosidase, 150
antibiotics
    calcification and, 35–36, 63
    during lactation, 70
    prescribed by dentist, 107, 129, 164
    prevention of tooth decay and, 111
    sugar in, 100
apical foramen, 30–31, 86
Aquafresh toothpaste, 152, 153
Aristotle, 13
arsenic, 198
arthritis, 112
ascorbic acid. *See* vitamin C
Australopithecus, 10
autism, 199, 214, 217

B
baby teeth. *See* deciduous teeth
bad breath, 131
baking soda, 145, 147, 193
barber-surgeons, 15
Bass, Charles C., 157
bicarbonate of soda, 145, 147, 193
bite splint, 183
Black, Green Vardiman, 21
bleeding gums, 58, 129–131
blood analysis, 184–185
body burden, 200, 226
Boer War, 22
braces. *See* orthodontics
breastfeeding, 42, 44, 67–70, 73–74
Brtitish Dental Association, 23
brushing. *See* tooth brushing
buccal surface, 29

Burke, Edmund, 18
B vitamins, 58–59, 69, 202

C
cadmium, 64, 198, 201, 203
caffeine, 64, 203
calcification
    described, 33–34
    birth trauma and, 34–35
    childhood illnesses and, 37
    fluoride and, 36
    genetics and, 37
    nutrition and, 38–42
    syphilis and, 36–37
    tetracycline and, 35–36
    trauma and, 38
calcium
    importance of, 38–40, 59
    interference with, 56, 64, 76
    in milk, 67, 79
    in premature babies, 66
    sources of, 39, 74
    in teeth, 38–40
calcium carbonate, 148
calcium glycerophosphate, 148
calculus, 124, 150, 152, 154, 155
cancer, 134, 162, 167, 169–171
canines, 28
caoutchouc, 21
carbohydrates, 97
caries. See tooth decay
cavities, 105
    See also tooth decay
celiac disease, 76
Celsus, Aulus Cornelius, 13–14

cement, 33
cetylpyridinium chloride, 148
chapatti, 41
chelation
    about, 213–218
    supplements for, 206, 219–227
chewing gum, 101, 154
chicken pox, 37
childhood illnesses, 37
Chirurgia Magna (de Chauliac), 15
chlorhexidine, 148–149, 151, 160
Chopra, Deepak, 177
chronic gum disease, 129
clenching of teeth, 127
coenzyme Q10, 137, 206
coffee, 64, 101, 102, 112, 203
Colgate Total toothpaste, 150, 154
colostrum, 67, 68
confectionery, 98
conservative dentistry, 26
contraceptives, 51, 70, 126, 163
Crest toothpaste, 153
crowded teeth, 46, 47, 82

D
dairy, 189–190
decay. See tooth decay
de Chauliac, Guy, 15
De Chirurgia (Abulcasis), 14
deciduous teeth
    described, 27–29
    abnormalities in, 81–82

accidental damage to, 85–86
at birth, 66–67
dentist and, 81
eruption of, 70–73
mixed dentition period and, 86–89, 92
thumb sucking and, 85
tooth decay in, 82–85, 102–103
DEHA (diethylhexyl), 190
dementias, 217
dental examinations, 162–169
dental floss, 156–158
dental history, 165
dentin, 31–33, 34, 85, 103, 105, 110
dentinogenesis imperfecta, 37
dentistry
    in antiquity, 12–14
    holistic, 3, 7–8, 51, 81, 83–85, 180–181
    in the Middle Ages, 14–18
    modern history of, 19–23
    profession of, 23–26
dentures, 12–13, 17, 21, 24
De Re Medicina (Celsus), 13–14
detox diet, 201–204
diabetes, 98–99, 108, 127, 188
diet. *See* nutrition
dietary guidelines, 187–196
dietary supplements, 136–137, 204–206
diet sheet, 185–186
di-indolylmethane (DIM), 220–221
dioxin, 190
disclosing tablets, 159
distal surface, 29
DMSA, 221
domiphen bromide, 149
drugs, pharmaceutical, 63
Dyer, Wayne, 177

E

eczema, 51, 63
EDTA, 219, 221–222
education, 26
Egyptians, 12
Elizabeth I, 16–17
enamel
    fluoride and, 115, 116
    sensitive teeth and, 3
    in structure of the tooth, 31–33, 34
    thumb sucking and, 85
    tooth decay and, 96, 103, 104, 105
    toothpaste ingredients and, 148
endocrine disruptors, 220–221
eruption cyst, 88
estrogenic esters, 175, 190
estrogens, 220–221
Etruscans, 12–13
Evans, Thomas, 21
exercise, 52, 177–178

F

Facussi, Nicol, 18
family meals, 80–81
fats, 57, 203
Fauchard, Pierre, 19

feng shui, 175
fetal alcohol syndrome (FAS), 65
fiber, 189, 202, 222–223
fight or flight response, 178
fish, 53, 57, 116, 201
fizzy drinks, 3, 93, 102, 109, 168
flossing, 156–158
fluoride
    potential hazards of, 36, 64, 114–115
    prevention of tooth decay and, 96, 104, 116–119
    in toothpaste, 120, 149–150
    topical, 32–33, 84, 89, 103, 104–105, 111, 119–121
    in water supplies, 117–118
fluorosis, 36, 92, 114, 115, 116
folic acid, 59
food additives, 65, 189
food labels, 77, 99–100
food sensitivities, 74, 76
food wrappings, 190
Foresight, 50, 51, 54, 62
Fox, Joseph, 20
free radicals, 218
French College of Surgeons, 18

G
gantrez, 150
garlic, 220
genetics, 37, 82, 96, 108, 125–126
German measles, 50, 51
gingivitis, 60, 123, 128, 130, 131, 149, 154
    See also gum disease
glucose oxidase, 150
gluten allergy, 76
Goodyear, Charles, 21
Gordon, Garry, 197, 213, 217, 221, 226
Gray, John, 177
Greeks, ancient, 13–14
Greenwood, John, 19
grinding of teeth, 127
gum disease
    described, 122–123
    causes of, 123–128, 205
    dentist and, 137, 162
    diagnosis of, 129
    nutrition and, 7, 127, 135–136
    during pregnancy, 60, 126
    progress of, 133
    signs of, 129–133
    tooth brushing and, 139
    types of, 128–129
gutta-percha, 21

H
Habsburgs, 45
hair analysis, 50, 62, 184
Haley, Boyd, 197, 198
Hamilton, David R., 207
Harris, John, 145
Hawkins, David, 209
headaches, 181–183
heavy metals
    chelation supplements for, 220–225

toxicity of, 197–202, 213–218
hemolytic anemia, 66, 67
Hepatitis A, 164
Herrick, Robert, 17
hexetidine, 151
Hippocrates, 13, 179–180
holistic dentistry, 3, 7–8, 51, 81, 83–85, 180–181
Homo erectus, 10
Homo habilis, 10
hormonal changes, 126
Howard, John, 113
Hunter, John, 19
hydrogen peroxide, 151
hydroxyapatite, 34
hypocalcification, 33–34, 35, 92
hypoplastic, 41

I
incisors, 28
iron, 55–56, 58, 59, 66
It's the Thought That Counts (Hamilton), 207

J
jaundice, 66, 67
jaws
    about, 42–44
    dysfunctions of, 85, 165, 166, 181–183
    shape of, 10, 44–48
    size of, 90, 94
juices, 74–75
juvenile delinquency, 108
juvenile periodontitis, 128

K
Klinghardt, Dietrich, 214

L
lactation, 69–70
L-ascorbic acid, 223
laughing gas, 21
lead
    chelation supplements for, 220, 223
    toxicity of, 62–63, 197, 198, 200, 216, 218
Levy, Thomas, 223
lichen planus, 167
lingual surface, 29
Listerine, 151
loose teeth, 133

M
malic acid, 223
malocclusions, 47, 68, 69
measles, 37
meat, 189–190, 194
medical history, 163–165
medications, 126–127
meditation, 177
menopause, 126
mercury
    in amalgam fillings, 20, 53, 61–62, 70, 213–214
    in baby medicine, 72
    chelation supplements for,

220–225
in pesticides, 63
toxicity of, 174, 197–201, 213–217
mesial drift, 94
mesial surface, 29
metronidazole, 129
micro-mercurialism, 214–215
microwave ovens, 61
migraines, 181–182
milk, 39, 56, 68, 78–79
milk teeth. See deciduous teeth
Millar, W. B., 97
minerals, 55–56, 59–60, 66, 189
mixed dentition period, 86–89, 92
molars, 28–29, 30, 87–88, 103, 117
Moro reflex, 43
mouth cancer, 162, 167, 169–171
mouth ulcers, 134, 159, 160, 206
mouthwashes, 121, 159–160
Mouton, Pierre, 19

N
National Health Service, 24, 95, 173
The Natural History of the Human Teeth (Hunter), 19
nicotine, 51–52, 64
   See also smoking; tobacco
nitrous oxide, 21
normal occlusion, 44–45

nutrition
   calcification and, 38–42
   detox diet, 201–204
   dietary guidelines for, 187–196
   gum disease and, 7, 127, 135–136
   health and, 2, 4–5, 170, 171
   high-protein diets, 42
   high-roughage diets, 41–42
   during lactation, 69–70
   organic foods, 52, 60, 65, 75, 76–77, 80, 190, 201
   preconception and, 52
   during pregnancy, 54–60, 82
   prevention of tooth decay and, 108, 111–112
   stress and, 179–180
   sugary snack foods and, 102
   teenagers and, 93, 128
   whole food diet, 52, 111, 187–188
nutritional counseling, 184–187
Nutrition and Physical Degeneration (Price), 4–5, 46–48

O
obstructive sleep apnea (OSA), 68–69
occlusal surface, 29
onions, 202–203
Oral-B toothpaste, 150
oral hygiene. See flossing; tooth brushing
organic foods, 52, 60, 65, 75,

76–77, 80, 190, 201
orthodontics, 85, 89–91, 94
osteoblasts, 43, 57, 58
osteoclasts, 43, 88
osteomalacia, 41
osteomyelitis, 12
oxalic acid, 42

P
pacifiers, 83, 102
pain, 31, 109–110, 132
Palmer, Brian, 68–69
papain, 152
Pare, Amboise, 15
Parmly, Levi Spear, 156–157
Pauling, Linus, 205, 223
penicillins, 129
periodontal disease. *See* gum disease
periodontal fibers, 30, 72
periodontitis, 123, 129, 130, 132
  See also gum disease
pharmaceutical drugs, 63
pica, 54
plaque
  fluoride and, 114, 116
  gum disease and, 123–125
  sugar and, 96–97, 100, 102
  tooth brushing and, 138–140, 142
  tooth decay and, 104, 105
  toothpaste ingredients and, 147, 149, 150, 154
plaster of Paris, 21
plastic, 190

Pliny the Elder, 14
postnatal care
  breastfeeding and, 42, 44, 67–70, 73–74
  feeding and, 74–81
  teeth and, 66–67
  teething and, 70–73
posture, 178
potassium nitrate, 152
Power vs. Force (Hawkins), 209
preconceptual care, 49–52
pregnancy
  dangers in, 61–65
  diet and, 54–60, 82
  holistic dentistry and, 53–54
  teeth and, 60, 126
  X-rays and, 53, 61
pre-molars, 28
prenatal care. *See* pregnancy
preservatives, 65, 189, 203
prevention, 26, 96, 110–113
Price, Weston A., 4–5, 46–48, 49, 50, 58, 179, 201
primitive man, 9–11
produce, 193–194, 201–202
proteins, 56–57
pulp, 31, 86, 105
purées, 75–78
pus, 132
pyorrhea, 137
pyrophosphates, 152

Q
quantum physics, 207

R

rampant tooth decay, 107–108, 109
receding gums, 131–132
red gums, 131
Rembrandt toothpaste, 152
remineralization, 105, 148, 150
Revere, Paul, 20
rheumatic fever, 163–164
rhubarb, 42, 76
rickets, 27, 41
Romans, ancient, 13–14
roots, 30, 33
Royal Army Dental Corps, 23
rubber, 21

S

salt, 52, 80, 188, 192
sanguinarine, 152–153
SBE (subacute bacterial endocarditis), 163
scaling, 14
scarlet fever, 37
scurvy, 7, 58, 136
Secundus, Caius Plinius, 14
selenium, 59, 203, 224
sensitive teeth
   causes of, 110
   fizzy drinks and, 3, 110, 168
   fluoride and, 116, 121, 150, 156
   tooth structure and, 33
serial extractions, 90–91
Shears, Elizabeth and Curtis, 192
Sheffield, Washington, 145

smoking
   body burden and, 201, 203
   gum disease and, 125, 137
   having children and, 51–52, 64, 70
   mints and, 101
   mouth cancer and, 170
Social Adjustment Rating Scale, 176
sodium lauryl sulphate, 153
sodium tripolyphosphate, 153
solid foods, 78–80
spina bifida, 59
spinach, 42, 58, 76
sprouts, 77–78, 194
stannous fluoride, 153
stress
   acid response and, 112
   acute ulcerative gingivitis and, 23, 128–129
   disease and, 173, 180–181
   environmental, 173–175
   gum disease and, 126, 128, 205
   lichen planus and, 167
   nutritional, 179–180
   pain threshold and, 109–110
   physical, 177–178
   psychological, 175–177
strontium acetate, 153
strontium chloride, 153
sugar
   in baby medicines, 72, 100
   consistency of, 102
   diet and, 4, 9, 93, 188, 192
   frequency of consumption and, 100

mercury and, 202
mixed dentition stage and, 89
in preconceptual diet, 52
tooth decay and, 82–83, 89, 96–104
supplements, 136–137, 204–206
swollen gums, 131
syphilis, 36–37

T
tartar, 124
teenagers, 93, 128
teeth
   described, 27–29
   at birth, 66–67
   color of, 91–92
   composition of, 34
   crowding of, 46, 47, 82
   eruption of, 71
   loose teeth, 133
   mixed dentition period, 86–89, 92
   molars, 28–29, 30, 87–88, 103, 117
   during pregnancy, 60, 126
   pre-molars, 28
   replanting of, 92–93
   sensitivity of, 3, 33, 110, 116, 121, 150, 156, 168
   structure of, 29–33
   teething stage, 70–73
   transplanting of, 18, 19
   wisdom teeth, 29, 94, 134, 159

See also deciduous teeth; tooth decay
tetracycline, 35–36, 63, 70, 92
thalidomide, 63
thimerosal, 199
thumb sucking, 85
tinnitus, 183
TMJ (temporomandibular joint) syndrome, 164, 181–183
tobacco, 125, 170
   See also nicotine; smoking
toothbrushes, 140–144
tooth brushing, 138–140
tooth decay
   abscesses and, 106–107
   acid production and, 100, 101–102
   cavities and, 105
   costs of, 95
   in deciduous teeth, 82–85, 102–103
   early stages of, 104–105
   pain and, 109–110
   prevention of, 110–113
   rampant tooth decay, 107–108, 109
   role of sugar in, 82–83, 89, 96–104
   during teenage years, 93
   transmission of, 108–109
tooth-drawers, 15–16
tooth enamel. *See* enamel
tooth fairy, 88
toothpastes
   fluoride in, 120, 149–150
   history of, 144–145

    ingredients of, 146–155
    manufacturers of, 96, 150, 152, 153
    types of, 155–156
toothpicks, 141, 160
trench mouth, 23, 128–129
triclosan, 154
Truman, Edwin, 21

V
vaccine, anti-decay, 111
van Leeuwenhoek, Antony, 17–18
Vigo, Giovanni, 15
Vincent's infection, 23, 128–129
visual display units (VDUs), 61
vitamin C
    about, 58, 136, 196
    contraceptive pill and, 51
    gum disease and, 58, 136, 205–206
    L-ascorbic acid and, 223
    mouth ulcers and, 134
    scurvy and, 7, 58, 136
    sources of, 74
Vitamin C, Infectious Diseases and Toxins (Levy), 223
Vitamin C and the Common Cold (Pauling), 205
vitamins
    B vitamins, 58–59, 69, 202
    healthy diet and, 189
    during pregnancy, 55–56, 57–59
    vitamin A, 57–58
    vitamin D, 40–41, 56

    See also vitamin C
vulcanite, 21

W
Wadsworth, H. N., 141
Washington, George, 19
Wells, Horace, 21
whole food diet, 52, 111, 187–188
wisdom teeth, 29, 94, 134, 159
wood points, 160
Wright, Jonathan, 221

X
X-rays, 53, 61, 90
xylitol, 154–155

Z
Zendium toothpaste, 150
zeolite, 224–225
zinc citrate, 155